AN
UNCOMPLICATED
LIFE

ALSO BY PAUL DAUGHERTY

Chad: I Can't Be Stopped
Fair Game

AN UNCOMPLICATED LIFE

A Father's Memoir of His Exceptional Daughter

PAUL DAUGHERTY

wm
WILLIAM MORROW
An Imprint of HarperCollinsPublishers

HarperCollins books may be purchased for educational, business, or sales promotional use. For information please e-mail the Special Markets Department at SPsales@harpercollins.com.

A hardcover edition of this book was published in 2015 by William Morrow, an imprint of HarperCollins Publishers.

FIRST WILLIAM MORROW PAPERBACK EDITION PUBLISHED 2015.

Designed by Jamie Lynn Kerner

Library of Congress Cataloging-in-Publication Data has been applied for.

ISBN 978-0-06-235995-7

15 16 17 18 19 ov/rrd 10 9 8 7 6 5 4 3 2

To Jillian, whose story resonates to all who hope

CONTENTS

Introduction   1
1   Praying Out Loud   10
2   Paul and Kerry   24
3   Kerry   41
4   Therapy   50
5   Dying to Breathe   61
6   Kelly   75
7   The First Angel   83
8   Jillian   91
9   Nancy   104
10 The Battleground of Dreams   119
11 Homework   131
12 The Coffee Song   145
13 The Two-Wheeler   156
14 Sometimes   167
15 Cymbidium Orchids Under the Porch Light   177
16 Kelly   192
17 An Appropriate Education   206
18 Belonging   219

19	Jillian and Ryan	225
20	I Hope You Dance	239
21	Missy and Tommy	252
22	College	261
23	In the Swing	267
24	Sometimes, We Drove	280
25	Dave Bezold	286
26	The Team	294
27	Jillian Turns 21	307
28	Testing	313
29	In Love and Moving Out	323
30	One More Drive	335
31	Vanuatu	340
32	Moving Day	352
33	Number 47	358
34	A Dream	363
Epilogue	Jillian and Ryan Get Engaged	366
	Acknowledgments	373

AN
UNCOMPLICATED
LIFE

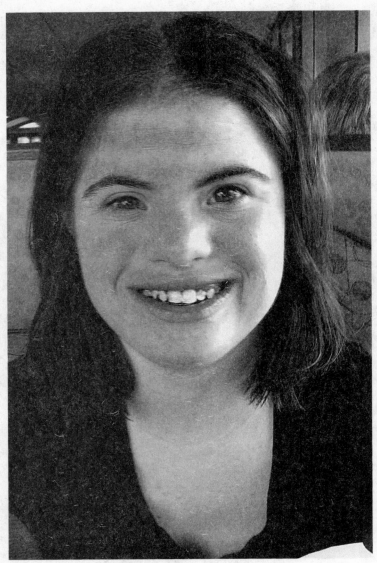

Jillian Phillips Daugherty.

INTRODUCTION

I wide bike."

This is a story about a dream and a child and the progress of each. It starts on our driveway in early spring.

Jillian Daugherty straddles a comically tiny two-wheeler that, against considerable odds and long-held perceptions, she intends to ride. She is 12 years old and prone to doing what all kids do. She's going to try to ride it.

Jillian has seen the neighborhood kids riding their bikes. More important, she has seen her brother, Kelly, who is older by three years, use his bike to breach the boundaries of the yard. Jillian idolizes Kelly, and she assumes she can do whatever he does so she has determined that mastering a two-wheeler will be the next frontier.

"Wide bike," she'd announced a few months earlier.

"What?" Eight years of speech therapy, and the r's still emerge as w's.

"I wide bike. Like Kelly."

It's a childhood rite of passage. Leaning to ride a bike is an afternoon of a parent steadying you and teaching you, holding you until you find your balance and your way, then letting you go. Unless you have Down syndrome. Then it's a little more complicated.

"Um, well . . ."

"I can do it," Jillian says. This would not be negotiable.

In the lengthy catalog of "Things Kids with Down Syndrome Probably Won't Do," managing a two-wheeled bike is somewhere between memorizing the dictionary and commanding a rocket ship. These children aren't sufficiently coordinated, and they don't have the balance. They are at risk of hurting themselves. And so on.

But my wife, Kerry, and I are hopelessly naïve or overly optimistic or both so we don't see the odds of Jillian's crashing to be much shorter than they are for any other kid. If she falls, she'll spit on the hurt and try again. This isn't the first time we've given a wide berth to our daughter's ambitions.

"Okay," we tell her. "When the weather warms up, we'll get you a bike."

"Tomorrow?" Jillian wonders.

A few months later, I am grasping the back of the bicycle seat lightly, as if I'm cradling a newborn. Jillian is tightly clenching the handlebars as a blue-perfect spring morning had summoned us to try again.

We'd been working at this for two months, at least. Jillian, being Jillian, had banged into this two-wheeled business with both feet. And both knees, both elbows and a forehead or two. It was like cracking a code or something in an effort to acquire the subtleties of balance and the blunt force of strength needed to keep the bicycle upright and beneath her.

Every day, I'd drag poor Jillian out to the long common asphalt drive we share with three other houses. I'd help her up, get her started and hold the back of her seat as she began pedaling.

Maybe this would be the day.

"You ready, superstar?"

"Yep."

Her bike looks like something a circus clown would use to chase elephants around a ring. It has wheels no more than a foot high, and a frame you could fold up and carry in your back pocket. It is small because so is Jillian. She's not quite 4 feet tall and weighs maybe 60 pounds. The helmet she's wearing drapes her head like a cheap slipcover. If Jillian looks down or to the side or in any direction other than perfectly straight ahead, the helmet pitches and yaws accordingly.

At the moment, Jillian sits in the seat, straight as a ruler.

"Dad, do you have me?" Jillian asks.

My fingertips own a tentative hold on the back edge of the bicycle seat. Jillian's audacity doesn't prevent her anxiety. "I have you," I say. "I will always have you."

WE'RE ALL CONNECTED.

I don't mean that in a saccharine, greeting-card sense. We're joined by situation and geography and happenstance. What we do with the connections that occur defines who we become. We can't thrive alone. Fulfillment needs partners.

Jillian Daugherty's life has been a happy conjoining of partners. Her story is about the power of a communal joining of hands and demonstrates that we were each put here to benefit the other. Three years after starting this project, this is what I will take from it. We're only as good as the way we treat each other.

The telling of Jillian's story involves many people. They are ordinary folks moved to extraordinary goodness by a child they often met by chance. Their lives are as rich as my daughter's, and every bit as sad and joyous, burdened and heroic. Spurred by compassion or justice or simple decency, they all helped Jillian become Jillian. In return, Jillian offered a mirror to their goodness. They couldn't help but like what they saw. They have helped Jillian live. She has helped them live better.

This was a book achieved in fits and starts. Bursts of adrenaline writing, surrounded by weeks and months of inactivity. I write about sports for a newspaper. I also write a daily blog. The random nature of it all means I am at once free and shackled. I work at home, usually, so I don't have to waste time commuting or talking with co-workers or eating lunch. That's good. I'm also on call. Teams don't fire coaches between nine and five on weekdays. Networks don't think about my dinnertime when they schedule games. Writing about sports requires flexibility and a tolerance for airport security lines. Your definition of a workweek is determined by when the games occur: All the time.

I have written this book on scraps of paper in airport terminals, and on the Long Island Railroad, bound for Manhattan. I've scribbled notions over a western omelet, on a paper napkin pulled from a dispenser in a diner in suburban Washington, D.C. From a promontory on Angel Island in San Francisco Bay, I've watched as fog draped the Golden Gate Bridge in fine white linen. Then I've used a golfer's pencil and the back of a ferry schedule to write down some ideas.

I tried writing in a rented room, believing such a setting would provoke good words and thinking. It didn't. We own a small cabin 70 miles east of our home in suburban Cincinnati. It's hard in the middle of Amish country, where solidly flat Ohio yields to the pleasant heaves of Appalachia. I went there, believing big thoughts would emerge from the pastoral curves of the land. They didn't.

Inspiration comes when you're not looking. I found it while wandering the vast and unharnessed Superstition Mountains outside Phoenix, where it was easy to see endless possibilities and how they'd impacted Jillian's life. Every summer, my son and I visit the Blue Ridge Mountains of North Carolina. Traversing the spine of those ancient hills provoked thoughts of mortality and living in the moment as best we can. That birthed a chapter on savoring Jillian's small wins.

"Nothing survives," Jackson Browne sang, "but the way we live our lives."

I don't know Joel Meyerowitz or Buzz Bissinger, but I am in their debt. Meyerowitz photographs landscapes. I have two of his books, which are made up of photographs of Cape Cod, Massachusetts. Meyerowitz's photos do for me what Edward Hopper's work does for lovers of paintings. The pictures, one in particular, fill me with the sort of abiding love and melancholy longing so necessary to the telling of Jillian's story.

Bissinger is known as a tough-guy journalist, but he didn't come off that way in his book *Father's Day,* about a cross-country road trip with his son. Not just any son, but an adult son with mental disabilities since birth. Bissinger struggles with his role as Zach's dad, and with his guilt for having not done better by him. I know the feeling.

My wife, Kerry, was, is and always will be Jillian's first champion. Kerry is a woman of extraordinary will and foresight. Jillian's map emerged from Kerry's determination. My son, Kelly, has been Jillian's shoulder. His full appreciation of his sister's presence has helped to give her the confidence to thrive in what otherwise might have been an overwhelming world.

Jillian's family is not just bound by blood. She owns a vast nation of family. Never underestimate the power of people to do good. The network of people who have influenced Jillian's life could fill a map of the world.

This book is mostly Jillian's doing. It is her book, and it is to her credit that it never occurred to me her story was book-worthy. She was our kid, and we loved her. Was she special? Only in the way everyone's kid is special.

But as I started dusting the corners of where she'd been and who she'd touched, I recognized what a trip it had been.

I began talking to the people Jillian had connected with: Teachers and coaches. Fathers and mothers, daughters and sons. I made the rounds of Jillian's life and found lots of fur-niture moved. She had touched people. She'd affected anyone who'd given her a look-see.

I started remembering things and interviewing people. I realized Jillian's successes belonged to—and were owed to—people far beyond Jillian. I realized that sharing her story might call attention to the power of the human spirit. This isn't a book about Jillian's disability. It's about how her disability has enabled more fully her life and the lives of others, none more than my own. Jillian makes us feel good for having been there.

HALFWAY DOWN THE DRIVE, Jillian hits her stride on her tiny new bike. Something kicks in. Confidence, maybe. The knowledge that my hand is still on the back of her seat, even as my grip can't hold a pencil. She pedals faster.

"Dad . . . ?"

The driveway is a few hundred yards long, a safe distance from the street and a good place to meander. It's one of those suburban creations, at once welcoming and self-contained. The common drive allows you to be close to your neighbors—or apart from them. It's what you make of it.

We didn't choose this house for its driveway. Not entirely. But we embraced it soon enough. No bouncing balls would find their way into the path of a car. Kelly was a year old when we moved in. Jillian has lived here always. Until we got this bicycle, her world was the house and the yard. Now it's about to be something more.

"Dad . . . ?"

This is a book about letting go. Kerry and I have prepared for this moment, and for all the moments to come. From the day we said hello to Jillian, we began to say goodbye. It's what parents do, with all our children. We love them so they can leave. Each parental act is a gentle palm in the small of the back. At some point, if we're lucky, our desire becomes their experience. We teach, we steady, we hold. And then we let go of the bicycle seat.

Even if our children have a disability. Maybe especially so.

"Dad? Are you back there?"

I am but a little less so. Letting go is a brisk walk, then a jog. It takes everything you have. When it's your daughter and she has Down syndrome, it takes more than that. More than everything.

I shift into a light trot so I can keep up with Jillian as she gains speed. I curl an index finger beneath the back of the seat.

"Dad, am I doing it?" she asks. "Am I wide?"

Jillian pedals harder. The bike wobbles, attuned to her uncertainty. I keep an airy hold, as much as is needed.

"I have you," I say. And then I don't.

The end of the driveway is just up ahead. So is the beginning of something brand new. Jillian says something, but it is lost in the breeze. I am standing halfway down the drive, hands stuffed in my pockets, no longer attached to my daughter's bike, trying not to cry. Jillian ker-bumps off the curb and onto the street, laughing.

She is a blueprint for how the rest of us can be. She lives the lessons we give.

I say this not because Jillian is my daughter, but because it is so. Jillian is a soul map of our best intentions.

She has affected everyone who has taken the time to see her. Seeing isn't easy. It requires participation. It implies understanding. Seeing is a mandatory swatch of the human fabric. It invokes a civil right. *Do not judge me on what I look like. See me for who I am.*

The narrow day-to-day confines of who we are don't always advance the promise of who we can be. Occasionally we need guidance. It doesn't have to be a bolt of lightning or wisdom from a book. It can come in the form of a child whose initial presence was terrifying and overwhelmingly sad and who just now hopped from the curb on the two-wheeler she was never expected to ride.

"Dad," Jillian said. "I wide!"

WHAT SORT OF PEOPLE do you like?

Who asks you in and prompts you to stay? People who are

kind, probably. Kindness is at the center of all we hope to be. If you are kind, you are trusting and trustful. You don't judge. Judging implies superiority. It makes people uncomfortable.

Chances are, you appreciate people without guile. They see the best in you. They're not looking for something beyond what the relationship suggests. They put you at ease. You never worry about agendas with guileless people. They're easy to be around.

People whose hearts are big and open. You like them. You like being around them because of the joy they make and the vulnerability they express. Their obvious frailties prompt your confidence. Big-hearted people own a broader humanity. They accept. Their wide soul berth inspires you.

Your best friend might aspire as well. He will say, "Why not?" He might fashion those Why-Not's into reality because he honors himself by always doing his best. He doesn't want to let you down, either. That's part of it. He knows how to be happy, and to make others happy.

You are drawn to people with patience because you've felt the power of the patience others have shown you. You like humility because you've been humbled. You appreciate grace because it's so often lacking.

What if you could know someone who has all that?

Jillian's heart is an uncomplicated place. It's hardwired to her brain. What Jillian feels, she mostly says. We can be in the car, or at lunch, or watching TV. We can be just about anywhere, when Jillian will launch a sigh and a smile, just because and apropos of nothing.

"I love my life," she'll say. "I just love my life."

CHAPTER 1

Praying Out Loud

After great pain a formal feeling comes;
The nerves sit ceremonious like tombs.
—EMILY DICKINSON

Jillian emerged in a rush, a week early and without labor. She was a watermelon seed between thumb and forefinger. She couldn't wait to be born.

Her brother's birth had taken fourteen hours. Half a day to make up his mind, and even then Kelly arrived without commotion. He didn't cry. He was curious. His saucer-eyes cased the delivery room. So, this is life.

Jillian burst from Kerry on October 17, 1989. In full throat, arms flailing, legs squirming, eyes seeking every possibility. Here I am. She was rockets-red-glare from the start.

I was a sports columnist for the *Cincinnati Post*, and I was in San Francisco for the World Series when Kerry called to say she was in labor and heading to the hospital. The San Francisco Giants and Oakland A's would have to wait. I caught the red-eye at about 11:00 p.m. West Coast time. Jillian was born before I left California airspace.

I got to the airport in Cincinnati at about 6:00 a.m. and called the hospital from baggage claim.

"How's the baby?" I asked Kerry.

"Great," she said.

"You?"

"Fine."

"Girl, right?"

"Girl," said Kerry.

My wife of six years had given birth to a girl. My girl. Daddy's girl. Pink dresses and tea parties. Cymbidium orchids beneath the porch light, warmed by moon glow and kisses after the first big dance. A stately walk of a lifetime, down a church aisle. I would get to do that now.

I fairly floated to baggage claim. The soliloquy from the musical *Carousel* played in my head:

> *You can have fun with a son*
> *But you gotta be a father to a girl.*

A few hours later, I began my negotiations with God.

Kerry was sitting up in bed when I arrived at Good Samaritan Hospital in Cincinnati, Room 507. Your wife never looks more beautiful than on her wedding day—unless it's in the hours after she has given birth. Kerry looked to have been kissed by the sun and the moon.

"Okay?" I asked.

Yes, she was. She was fine and radiant. She held Jillian

in her arms, covered in a pink blanket. One eye, brown and almond-shaped, peaked out from under the swaddling. An arm no bigger than an oak twig, a fist the size of a golf ball. A pinky finger, curled slightly and strangely inward, as if it were arthritic.

"I'm your dad," I said.

My wife's friend Gayle had taken her to the hospital. She was there when Jillian was born. "She's perfect," Gayle said. As the nurse stitched her up, Kerry filmed the goings-on.

"No Down syndrome?" she had asked Gayle.

"No Down syndrome."

It was not an offhand question.

For nine months, we had kept seeing people with Down syndrome. We'd noticed them, where we never had before. At the mall, at the movies, at the grocery store. Here and there. We'd spent 15 days in Europe in June. At a café in the French coastal town of Arromanches, a woman sipped coffee in an outdoor courtyard while she held her baby, who had Down syndrome.

"It doesn't mean anything," I'd said to Kerry that day.

Kerry was 34 years old when Jillian was conceived. We worried about that, but not much. Kerry was healthy. She'd emerged from Kelly's birth with no complications. She had been preparing for this moment her whole life. Being a wife and mother was who she always wanted to be. She didn't drink alcohol in college because she knew she wanted to have kids. During her pregnancy with Jillian, Kerry left the room when Kelly and I were gluing a model airplane. For nine months, she ate nothing stronger than toast.

My mother had been ignorant of the prenatal precautions

we take for granted now and smoked and drank while she carried me. I was born six weeks early, weighed barely four pounds and spent my first week in an incubator. Jillian faced none of that. She emerged robust and curious and pink.

We had scheduled an amniocentesis for the 20-week mark of Kerry's pregnancy. A woman of 35 isn't old to bear children, but she's not young either. The potential was there for disability. We also wanted to know the sex, so Kelly could become familiar with his younger sibling before her birth. Two nurses explained to us the procedure: They'd do an ultrasound to see where Jillian was in the womb. They'd note the position of the amniotic sac. Then they would insert a needle and withdraw a small amount of amniotic fluid. That would be tested for a few days and would tell them if Jillian had Down syndrome, or any number of other disabilities.

Medical technology has advanced since that time. Blood tests, carried out during a woman's first trimester of pregnancy, are safer and less invasive. Amniocentesis can cause miscarriages and generally isn't performed until the second trimester, when aborting a pregnancy can be more traumatic and harder to obtain. New science will provide prospective parents with a scientific clarity we didn't have in 1989. It will also open a Pandora's box of moral choices.

In 2010, a woman had a one in 733 chance of carrying a child with Down syndrome. Close to 90 percent of pregnant women who receive the diagnosis choose to abort. What would new tests offering greater accuracy do to that statistic?

"Will babies with Down syndrome slowly disappear?" wondered Brian Skotko, a fellow in genetics at Children's Hospital in Boston.

We choose to celebrate some of our differences now. Will we choose also to eliminate others? Who decides?

This wasn't an issue in the spring of 1989 as Kerry lay on a doctor's office table, awaiting the amnio. I was there to lend moral support and manly courage to the proceedings. No woman should have to endure that alone. I was there, quietly strong, at least until the nurses described the procedure. Then I went weak in the legs and folded at the waist. The room turned.

The nurses caught me, one on each arm, and led me from the room. I had to take all that manly moral support out to the waiting area, where I spent some time fanning myself and recovering from the trauma of hearing about the procedure. After a while, everyone came out.

"Well?" I asked.

"They couldn't do it," Kerry said.

"Why not?"

"The baby was in the way."

Our baby girl's position in the womb made drawing the fluid dangerous. So they didn't. Several weeks later, Kerry had an ultrasound to learn the sex. It was a girl. We named her Jillian three months before she was born. We didn't know if the technicians who performed the procedure had seen anything to suggest to them the baby had Down syndrome. We still don't know. We've never asked.

We left the doctor's office unconcerned. Kerry laughed at all the "help" I'd been, and I went back to work.

Now, it's 19 weeks later, and I am holding my wife and our newborn briefly. I am going home to get Kelly so I can introduce him to his sister. "I'm your dad" is what I say again, as I walk out of Room 507 for the 30-minute drive home.

Jillian's birth was different for me than Kelly's. I was more ready to be a father. I'm not saying I wasn't daunted again. If the gravity of parenthood doesn't grip you every time, you shouldn't be in the game. But the weight felt lighter this time. I knew some things about being a parent. I knew the lay of the land.

Parenting is trial and error, no matter how long you do it. But I'd been to the big leagues once already. I'd hit the pitching.

I was more willing, too. Kerry had been full-bloom ready to be a mother when Kelly was born. I was very much riding shotgun. The prospect of fatherhood scared me, but not as much as I believed it would limit me.

We'd been married for more than three years when Kelly arrived. They were easy years. I woke up every morning next to my best friend, with whom I shared interests and passions. We had a small bungalow in Norfolk, Virginia, two hours from the mountains and 20 minutes from the beach. We did what we wanted, when we wanted. I liked the freedom and the companionship. I was reluctant to give that up.

We had a 60-pound shepherd-collie named Deja-Vu. Wasn't that child enough?

You don't realize that time shared with a baby is every bit as intimate as time shared alone together. At least I didn't. All I could think was "there go the weekends in the Shenandoahs."

As I walked in our front door to pick up Kelly, the phone was ringing. It was Kerry. She offered a low guttural moan like nothing I'd ever heard. "You need to come back now," she said. "The doctors think Jillian has Down syndrome."

There are days you remember always, for the weight of

their woe. I remember the day my mother downed 100 sleeping pills to ease her pain forever. I remember the day we put down our first dog, caressing her muzzle as the vet injected the lethal dose. And I remember this day, when the wife I'd left happy and glowing with a baby in her arms called to tell me our baby had Down syndrome.

After I left, a doctor Kerry had never seen had told her. He declared it in matter-of-fact tones. He proclaimed my daughter "floppy" in reference to her low muscle tone. He thought Kerry knew.

She called me immediately. I held the phone to my ear. "What?" I said.

At a moment like that, you want only to be told you misheard. You think, maybe it's a wrong number. There is another Kerry, and she is calling another Paul. It's all a big mistake. Has to be.

Kerry repeated the news.

"Oh, no," I said.

I don't know how other parents react to hearing that they have an imperfect baby. I've never asked. I dealt with that moment by making perfectly logical, impossible demands. I didn't want a miracle. That wouldn't be enough.

I started my negotiation with God.

"Take me," I said.

I pleaded with God because at that moment, no one else would do. A life for a life, right now, straight up. I am 31 years old. I have seen things, felt things, done things. Life has made its mark on me. Jillian is the first day of spring.

I am not especially religious, but I am religious enough to believe this was not a random act perpetrated upon my little girl. Jillian, my daughter of six hours, has Down syndrome. A bum spin of the chromosomal wheel has produced the peculiar genetics that will rule her life.

I had a deal. What The Man had done, He could undo.

"Take me," I said.

Meanwhile, Kelly wouldn't be coming to see his sister just yet. I checked with the neighbor who was watching him, told her the black news, then got back in the car and returned to Good Samaritan Hospital.

This is how we change. It's not gradual. It comes in a flash and is beholden to events we can't foresee or control. Change is instant. Reacting is a lifetime. What must I have looked like to those passing me on the interstate? What's with that guy, crying and slamming his fists on the steering wheel, yelling to himself?

Take me. I was as insistent as I was irrational. This might be a negotiation, but the wiggle room was limited. In this profound instant of grief, I wanted what I wanted. "Don't do this to her. She's just a little girl. Take me. Make her better. Tell us the doctors are wrong. Don't do this to my little girl. Oh, god." Oh, God.

My mind was cottony as I made my way back to Room 507. Voices converged. I wasn't in a 12-by-12 private room anymore. I wasn't listening to one distinct voice across a space that suddenly had become as quiet as Sunday morning. My brain was layered in gauze. I couldn't discern the voice that came from the man—or is it a woman?—wearing the white scrubs and the stethoscope. I heard a crowd, as if we were at a ball game or a bar. Disbelief muffled everything.

"Things are so much better for these kids now . . ."

These kids?

I wanted to float to the top of the room. I wanted to fly away.

Just yesterday I was in a rental car, driving Highway 1 north of San Francisco. It was a golden autumn day. The blue of the Pacific and the velvety brown of the hills stretched for miles in front of me. Anything was possible.

I wished it were still yesterday and would be forever.

"We will get you all the information you need . . ."

I take Jillian in my arms again. I wonder if she feels different than she did an hour earlier. The weight of a newborn isn't measured in pounds because hope has no scale. Intellectually, I'm already making the turn to "what's next?" Emotionally, I have miles to go. I stare unblinking into the central moment of the rest of my life.

Jillian is wearing a pink gown and a white knit hat. She alternates between curious staring and soft sleep. The doctors say she weighs 6 pounds, 11 ounces, but she feels heavier. Joy is portable. It is born on the wind. Feeling good involves a sort of weightlessness. Joy travels well.

Grief stays put. It is resolute, something to be carried until your back bends.

Lift up your hearts. Lay down your burden.

That first day, Jillian weighed a million pounds. We all did.

I held Jillian in my arms, ponderously.

"She's beautiful, Ker'," is the best I could do.

Words aren't solace. Nothing is. Wisdom comes later and is properly hard-earned. First, we cry.

In the haze, Kerry tried to rationalize. She returned to her premonitions during pregnancy. "I thought the whole time it might not be true," she said. "But I knew. I did."

Official results from genetic testing would take a few weeks to confirm the initial diagnosis. On this first day, the doctors were observing Jillian's pinky fingers that curled in. I looked at the medical chart hanging from the bottom of the hospital bed. "Simian creases on the palms" someone had written. I took Jillian's hand in mine. I turned it over, palm upward. Horizontal lines ran the breadth of her tiny palm. I looked at my own palm. Different lines. At moments like that, fear assumes its own visceral presence. It becomes part of you. Eyes, ears, mouth. Heart, lungs, blood. Fear.

I go home for a second time to pick up Kelly and bring him to the hospital and introduce him to his little sister.

By mid-morning, Kerry's parents arrive at the hospital from their home in Pittsburgh. She tells them. Sid Phillips, her father, says nothing. He sits down, mulling it. We wonder if he knows what Down syndrome is. Kerry's mother, Jean, covers her in a hug. Both cry silently. "Don't cry, Mom," Kerry said. "I don't want Kelly to think there's anything wrong with his sister."

Kelly sits in a chair, holding a stuffed bear meant for Jillian. He is three years old. "You have a cool little sister" is what I tell him.

I call my parents in Florida for the second time that day. On that first day, heartbreak runs in a continuous loop.

"I need you to sit down," I tell my stepmother. I break the news.

"I'll have to call you back," she says. Later she will tell me she spent that afternoon meditating and had a vision of Jesus, holding Jillian in His arms and telling her everything would be fine. But for now, my stepmother has to get off the phone and cry.

My dad gets on. "Who does she look like?" he asks. The most beautiful and personal moments of a lifetime can die in a hospital room. It was all he could think to ask.

"Dad, she doesn't look like anyone."

And so it went. Kerry's parents left after a while. They took Kelly back to our house. I took a shower in the hospital room. I needed something to be washed away. I wasn't sure what it was. Guilt, maybe. Regret. Sadness. Surely, sadness. The water felt like tears from a faucet.

The negotiation with God was a failure. I was still here. Jillian still had Down syndrome. Figuring I had nothing to lose at this point, I hurled invectives like fastballs at the Almighty. A just God would not have allowed this. So screw Him.

At 8:00 p.m., ABC sports broadcaster Al Michaels was in the television booth at Candlestick Park, setting up the first pitch of the first game of the 1989 World Series. Then the earth shook all around him. Michaels nearly fell from his stool. The earthquake would delay the Series an entire week. People died. Journalists would work by candlelight. They would feel their way, wondering if the earth was done quaking. A friend covering the Series told me it felt as if the Bay Area—disconnected, broken, devastated—was the last, worst place on earth.

"You have no idea," he said.

"Yes," I replied. "I do."

It was 2:00 a.m. when Kerry's crying woke me up. The heartbreak in that small space in time seemed irreversible. There was nothing to do but cry. Kerry hadn't cried all day. Every time she wanted to, some counselor would come in. She didn't want to upset Sid, Jean and Kelly, either, but they were back at our house now.

"I don't know what we're going to do, Paul," Kerry says.

I knew what we were going to do. But only for that moment. I didn't know it then, but I would learn: When you have a child with a disability, all that matters is now. What can you do this minute, this hour, this day? The circle is as tight and dense as a fist. Yesterday is meaningless, tomorrow is overwhelming. Now is the only thing you can do something about.

With one hand, I rub my wife's red and swollen face and push the hair from her eyes. With the other, I take her arm.

"Come on," I say.

I pull her up slowly. Grief weighs. Kerry had spent nine months adding weight. Some 24 hours earlier, she'd shed it, gloriously. Now, she feels leaden and a little less alive. With both hands, I help her from the bed.

"Let's go."

At 2:00 a.m. a hospital ward comes with its own contradictions. Quiet and too quiet. Hopeful and hopeless, peaceful and full of dread. All at once. Nurses with reassuring words, delivered in patronizing tones. Brightly lit corridors remove all the gray areas and prevent you from hiding your terror. They illuminate your sadness and hope equally.

We leave Room 507 with its mocking array of balloons, cards and flower arrangements, and walk down the hall. On the left is a window and through that window is a nursery full of newborn babies.

"Jillian Daugherty," I say to a nurse.

Nothing in life is better than birth. Hope knocks anew. You might have screwed up everything else in your life, but when your baby arrives, your soul's calendar flips to a fresh page. This feeling might not last forever. It could disappear the moment you leave the womb of the maternity ward. In that first moment, though, it's there. Plain as a sunrise. You have a new purpose.

And now?

The nurse brings our child. She is wrapped deeply in her pink blanket. Someone has attached a pink bow to the wisps of her soft brown hair. Jillian is sleeping. I give her to Kerry. "It's going to be okay," I say. Whether I believe that or not doesn't matter. I need to say it. Kerry needs to hear. "Our little girl is going to be all right."

Kerry takes the miracle and holds it lightly. Love is weightless. "I know," she says.

There are things you learn along the way, things that help you deal with that awful moment and, eventually, to understand that it wasn't so awful. Having a child with a disability is like having a life coach you didn't ask for. You realize that perspective is a blessing that's available to anyone who seeks it. Or has it forced upon him.

The miracle of an imperfect child is the light she casts on your own imperfections. After a time, she will teach you far more than you will teach her, and you will discover that "normal" comes with a sliding scale.

You realize a kind of love you never knew you had. Nothing magical that happens, from the first tying of shoes to the first solo flight on a two-wheeler to the first time she shows us her paycheck, is ever again assumed. Life's everyday worthwhiles take their proper place in the happiness queue.

The potential for kindness becomes self-evident and the universal need for compassion abides.

Twenty-four years later, if Kerry and I know anything, we know this: We're better human beings for knowing Jillian. She was put here to make us better people. That's the all of it.

I have forgotten lots of things about Jillian's life in the 24 years since that first day. Poignant, funny things. Things that made me rage. Snapshots of who she was becoming. I've relied on the better memories of others to color what's gray. I haven't forgotten that phone call, though. I've never again experienced the dark kaleidoscope of emotions encountered in those first 24 hours. I've never felt more alive. I've never wished more that I weren't.

Jillian was born October 17, 1989. It was the last bad day.

CHAPTER 2

Paul and Kerry

For us, there is only the trying.
The rest is not our business.
—T. S. ELIOT

I was six years old and in the second grade when my mother first tried to kill herself. I had just come home from school when I found her lying on the kitchen floor, blood from her opened wrists pooling on the linoleum.

"What do you want me to do?" I asked her.

My mother said something I didn't understand.

"What?"

This was 1964, and there was no 9-1-1 in those days. There were numbers in a phone book for doctors and ambulances and police, but I didn't know how to find them. I stumbled through another plea. "What can I do?"

I knocked on the door of the neighbor's apartment and rang the bell. No answer.

I returned to the kitchen. This was the first time I'd seen blood. "What do you want me to do?" I said again. Maybe my mother said "Call Dad," but I don't remember. I didn't know his work number anyway.

That's when I went out to play.

I don't remember the rest of the day. My dad must have come home fairly soon after that, and they must have gone to the emergency room. Someone sewed my mother's wrists. Later that night, my father woke me up.

"You saw your mother lying there and didn't do anything?"

"I didn't know what to do," I said weakly.

"So you went outside to play?"

For a long time after that, my mother's wrists were wrapped in bandages, and she would wear long sleeves to cover her arms. She looked sad, tired, disappointed, defeated.

"I didn't know what to do," I repeated.

That's when my dad told me what to do if something like this ever happened again. He was giving a six-year-old instructions on what to do the next time his mother tried to kill herself.

TWO YEARS LATER, WHEN I was in the fourth grade, my mother completed her task. We were living in a first-floor, garden-style apartment with a front door and a sliding glass door in the back. The day she died, both doors were locked. That day I got off the school bus, walked to the apartment and tried the front door. When I discovered it was locked, I went around to the glass door. I knocked on it, but I could tell my mother wasn't home. I sat in a chair on the porch and did my homework.

This was unusual, but not completely strange. Sometime before that, my mother had bought a handgun and shot a hole through the ceiling of our apartment. I didn't know why she did that. I've never asked. Doctors said she was "schizophrenic." She'd been put on medication.

"Who would you rather live with? Me or Mommy?" my dad had once asked me during an especially unhappy night.

"I love you both," I said.

Understanding something as complex as a flawed human brain is beyond most of us. It wasn't on my radar as a kid in elementary school. It wasn't even a concept. The times my mother checked into the "mental hospital" were explained to me as you might expect:

"Mom is sick. These people are going to make her well."

Well, okay. Who's going to make dinner?

WHEN YOU ARE A child, all you really want is no surprises. There ought to be a comforting sameness. Cake on birthdays. Sleepovers, dinner at six and no TV until the homework is done. The calculus of a kid's life should not be complex: Love, security and a place to go. And that place should be immovable so his world spins in a tight circle. Home is where you go that makes nowhere else matter. The monsters you see shouldn't be the ones that scare you.

My mother said she heard voices. She sometimes kept me home from school because she wanted the company. She was a loving mother, and we took long walks to the park, where she pushed me on the swings and laughed when I let her down quickly on the teeter-totter.

She loved the mountains of North Carolina. We'd spend a week in Montreat, a Presbyterian retreat 20 miles east of Asheville. The Rev. Billy Graham still lives in Montreat. It's a town of 250 people, tucked into a cove in the Black Mountains of the Blue Ridge. Calmness abides. Everyone says hello.

My mother and dad and I hiked the local Lookout Mountain. I ran up the hill, and they would pray to the Rev. Billy that I wouldn't take a header off the narrow trail. We hiked Grandfather Mountain, whose main attraction was a swinging bridge connecting twin peaks. When the wind blew—which it did all the time—the bridge swayed mightily, and I refused to cross it. To this day, my dad calls Grandfather Mountain "Chicken Peak" in my honor.

We'd venture into Asheville to eat at the S&W Cafeteria, where my "vegetables" were French fries and mashed potatoes. My mother was never happier than when she was roaming the spines of those ancient hills. Their beauty was cathartic.

After I'd been sitting on the porch for a while, my dad came home. The suicide note lay on the table in the dining nook. He read it as I sat on the porch, peering in. He put the note down. He opened the sliding glass door and held me for a long time.

"I think she's done it this time," he said.

My mother had left us by adding a hundred sleeping pills to her bloodstream—too many to pump away. She'd gone to her parents' apartment for the day. Mom died in her father's bed, in the apartment her parents shared in Washington, D.C. It was what she wanted. I don't know why she chose their apartment for the final goodbye. It didn't matter.

Memory is a con man. Time creates distance between what is

true and what we believe to be so. I remember my mother's death, though. It isn't a souvenir of recollection. It is part of who I am.

I am not fluent in the language of grief. The internal engines governing my emotions rarely crank up. I didn't cry much after my mother died. I was praised for that: "What a brave boy." It wasn't that. I wasn't brave. I repressed. I knew my mother wasn't coming back, and a part of me—a selfish, guilty, yet practical part—knew life would be hard after that. But it would never be so uncertain as it was when she was alive, when every day held the potential for love and terror in equal measure. I would be secure. My dad would ensure that. I would have a place to go, with no surprises. At the very least, the surprises wouldn't be the terrible kind I'd been used to.

THREE HUNDRED MILES TO the north and west, Kerry Phillips was eleven years old, almost four years older than I. She lived in Hopewell, Pennsylvania, 30 miles northwest of Pittsburgh, in the sort of fantasy world I knew only from television. Hopewell wasn't Mayfield where the Cleavers lived. And Sid and Jean Phillips weren't Ward and June. But the Cleaver ideal had a soul mate.

Kerry lived in a cocoon of family. She and her sister endured a babysitter exactly once. Every close relative lived within five miles of her front door, and the extended family could practically converse from its front porches. It was a time of middle-class prosperity, ensured by the huge and hulking Jones and Laughlin steel mill, which spread for seven miles along the Monongahela River, in nearby Aliquippa.

The area had benefited from the World War II demand for trucks and tanks and bullets, and after the soldiers came home, the mill remained busy, producing steel for automobiles, appliances and other accoutrements of the freshly unleashed American Dream. Union shops guaranteed the men would be paid well for their time. Moms didn't work outside the home. They fixed kids breakfast before sending them off to school. They filled metal Batman lunch boxes with peanut butter sandwiches and short thermoses with Kool-Aid. The kids came home to snacks. Houses were spotless. "I went through this phase in high school where I wanted Jell-O for breakfast," Kerry recalled. "Cut up in little squares, like you see in restaurants. My mother would make it in little squares and put it in a parfait glass for me."

At 4:00 p.m. or 5:00 p.m., or whenever Dad's shift at the mill ended, Mom had dinner on the table. The whole family ate together and talked about the day. Sundays were spent at church and at the homes of grandparents. Parents, siblings, aunts and uncles gathered to eat and live the family dream. It wasn't unusual for Kerry to spend all or part of her Sundays with 14 or 15 family members.

Summers were spent at the swim club. Jean would drop Kerry off at 10:30 in the morning for practice. Sid would pick her up at 4:00 p.m. After dinner, she would roam the safe, suburban avenues until the streetlights came on. That was the sign that it was time to go home.

Once a week, Kerry made the trip to Franklin Avenue in downtown Aliquippa, where her grandfather Oscar Barnhart owned a convenience store that had a soda fountain and a large candy counter. Oscar allowed his granddaughter one piece of free candy.

Oscar and his wife, Marie, lived within walking distance of the store. When Marie needed to get a message to Oscar at the store, she wrote a note and attached it to the family dog's collar. The pooch would amble the few blocks and present the note to Oscar. Before they owned the store, Oscar and Marie Barnhart taught school together in a one-room schoolhouse.

Kerry played flute in the Hopewell High marching band. She went to all of the football and basketball games, watching a classmate named Tony Dorsett break lots of records. Dorsett went on to a Hall of Fame career as a running back with the Dallas Cowboys.

Kerry says the home cocoon was so strong she never strayed. She never had the experience of being scared of a parent waiting for her when she missed curfew because she never missed curfew. She graduated from high school in 1972, yet never experimented with drugs, or knew anyone who did. Her dates were highly scripted: Movies, picnics or hanging at the local fast-food place, a strip-mall fixture called the Brighton Hot Dog Shoppe. Especially adventurous dates involved going to the Pittsburgh International Airport and watching airplanes arrive and depart.

MEANTIME, I'D LIVED IN the storm of my mother's schizophrenia.

In the days after she died, my dad and I returned to the apartment with the sliding-glass door. I took a few days off from school. We told everyone Mom had had a heart attack.

It was easier that way. My dad and I were making do. Jim Daugherty was steadfast. He had an eight-year-old son, he was all alone, his wife had just died in the most emotionally searing way, and he was heroic.

We were inseparable. "Wounded animals" my dad called us.

I got a key to the apartment. We tied it to a shoestring. I wore it under my shirt. Sometimes I twirled it in class. Other kids asked me what it was for. When I told them it was the key to where I lived, they were impressed. Having your own apartment key imparted a sort of freedom not seen among most fourth graders.

I was cool.

For my dad's peace of mind—and so I would have something to do after school besides be cool alone in my empty apartment—he hired a woman to watch me for a few hours until he could pick me up. Mrs. McKee lived just down the block from my best friend, walking distance from the elementary school.

Her duties mostly involved being there. If I couldn't go home to a real mom, I'd at least have an anchorage, a two-hour harbor where normalcy lived. Mrs. McKee offered the occasional snack. I'd drop my books and go out to play. No surprises.

Then one day, not long after we'd started this arrangement, I came to her house and found the door locked and the house silent. I went around back. That door was open so I went inside.

"Mrs. McKee?"

No answer.

"Mrs. McKee?"

"In here," she said. Mrs. McKee lay sobbing on her bed, wracked with pain from an ulcerous stomach.

"Are you okay, Mrs. McKee?" I asked.

She wasn't, of course. And I couldn't stay with her in the afternoons anymore.

My dad found someone else, and I shuttled just up the street, where Aline Alexander lived with her son and grandson. She wasn't my aunt, but I called her "Aunt Aline." She was a heavy smoker who was emphysemic. She was at home all day so Dad had found a new place to keep me in after-school orbit.

That is, until Aunt Aline was no longer able to keep me. She had lung cancer.

People kept disappearing.

AT 4:00 P.M. MOST weekdays, Kerry Phillips climbed the apple tree in her backyard in Hopewell. From there, she could see her dad's car coming up Harding Avenue. For 37 years, Sid worked for Aliquippa and Southern Railroad, in the Signal and Water Service Department. A&S was a subsidiary of the steel giant Jones and Laughlin, its railway spanning the seven-mile length of the mill. Sid served A&S as an electrician, a plumber or a welder. Whatever the day's work required.

The Phillips family—Sid, Jean, Kerry and her sister, Janis, two years her senior—sat down for dinner every night at 4:30 p.m. Family dinner was sacrosanct, and attendance was mandatory. For me, in the days when I was staying with Mrs. McKee, and then with Aunt Aline, in the afternoons, my dad would pick me up after work. Then most nights, we'd eat dinner at the apartment of my mom's parents. This was the same apartment where my mother had removed herself from all her earthly engagements.

Life wasn't terrible. My dad filled our loneliness with board games, and Pop-Tarts for breakfast. Eventually we began eating at home. Anything we could boil or slam into a toaster was suitable for consumption. We had season tickets to the Washington Redskins, a passion we shared with my mother's father. We drove Grandpa to the games. Each game he'd repay the gesture by buying me a program.

My dad made sure I owned what was left of our cocoon. Home was never an entirely safe harbor for either of us. Jim Daugherty offered the strength of a father and, as best as the gender allows, the touch of a mother.

"Waffles or pancakes?" he might ask as we circled the strange land of the supermarket.

"French toast," I'd answer.

Everything was frozen. Even now, my dad has the culinary skills of a college freshman. Anything that could be thawed and eaten, was. We were hungry men, living on Hungry Man.

A man with an eight-year-old son in tow doesn't have the luxury of grieving from the tragedy of a lifetime. That first winter, we went to basketball games. The Baltimore Bullets had a deal: Five dollars got you a game ticket and a seat on a Greyhound from the D.C. suburb of Langley Park to the arena in Baltimore. On Christmas night in 1966, my dad and I went to a game. He suggested it. We both needed something to be cheerful about. Today they call it father-son bonding. I don't know what we called it. It was equal parts love and desperation, faith and hopelessness. It was a mystery ride in a dark bus. It was all we had.

That night my father sat close to me in the darkness of the bus, closer than he ever would again. We talked. I wanted to know how Earl Monroe could dribble the basketball behind his back without bouncing it off his heel. I wanted to know why he called himself "The Pearl," a great leap of audacity in those less self-reverential times.

"Is Wilt Chamberlain the strongest man in the world, Dad?"

"I don't know," Dad answered.

"Can he beat up Wes Unseld?"

I wanted to know where the bus went after it dropped us off and before it picked us up again, how come Kevin Loughery shot so much and when my mother might be coming back. I wanted to know that.

"Why did Mom leave, Dad?"

He said she had an illness. It was nobody's fault. Especially not hers. This satisfied me then, and now. Betsy Daugherty *was* ill, to an extent not a lot of people in 1966 understood. Not the least of whom was the eight-year-old sitting on a dark bus on the way to a basketball game.

KERRY NEVER KNEW ANYONE who had a parent who died. She didn't know any latch-key kids, or any kids whose parents split up. Her world was Jell-O for breakfast, cut up in squares, in a parfait glass. Just so.

Sid Phillips also owned and operated an appliance repair business, Phillips Appliance Service. He was a one-man repair crew, mending everything from toasters to washing machines. He'd work his regular mill shift, come home, wash up, eat dinner with his family, then spend much of the rest of the evening on service calls.

The money paid for Kerry's and Janis's college educations, something that escaped Kerry until she graduated. "Now I'm done with Phillips Appliance Service," Sid announced shortly after Kerry got her diploma.

Times changed in Hopewell and in Aliquippa, but not until after Kerry Phillips had graduated and moved away. The mill shut down. Without J&L providing reliable, well-paying work, Aliquippa fell into disrepair. It became the place the TV networks used as the visual metaphor for the downfall of American manufacturing. White flight, a healthy drug culture, high unemployment and high crime took over and led to a kind of hopelessness. Once-vibrant Franklin Street, its businesses shuttered, became no place to be after dark. Oscar Barnhart sold the candy store and moved to Hopewell.

By 1982, Sid Phillips was forced to retire early from his job as a supervisor on the A&S Railroad. Until early 2014, he and Jean still lived comfortably in Hopewell, in the house Sid built shortly after he returned from World War II. Then they moved into a retirement community not far from Kerry and me. They've been married 69 years.

ABOUT A YEAR AFTER my mother died, Dad started dating. It had to be awkward for him, a 34-year-old widower suddenly back in the game. He joined Parents Without Partners, a social group for single parents seeking companionship. My mother's mother suggested it. Dad dated a few women but introduced me to only two of them. One was a divorcee with four children. The other was Elsye Allison, also divorced, raising twins. Jeff and Debra were 14 years old at the time.

At some point fairly early in the process, my dad shifted his attention to Elsye. Part of it was because he didn't want to inherit four of someone else's kids. Another part was, I liked Elsye better. After they'd been dating for six months or so, I asked out of the blue, the way nine-year-olds do, "Are you going to marry Mrs. Allison?"

"I don't know," my dad said. "I hadn't given it much thought."

He knew I needed a mother, though. I needed a softer voice telling me goodnight. Elsye was tough and no nonsense, yet she possessed a tenderness I sensed right away. I needed something else, too. I needed for the world to stop spinning. No more surprises. Someone to be there when I got off the school bus. Birthday cakes. I needed that more than anything.

My father married Elsye on June 1, 1968.

As I've grown up and raised my own family, I've come to appreciate what a dicey proposition a second marriage can be. Throw in the maelstrom of three kids, and survival odds are less than hopeful. I also wondered what my dad's biggest motivation was for marrying again. He doesn't like being alone. He wanted adult company. But how much of it was for me?

"I wanted a mother for you," he said not long ago. "And I got tired of being by myself."

Elsye and my dad bought a house in Bethesda, Maryland, that they could barely afford, for the security everyone had to have. In those days, Bethesda was a middle-class suburb of Washington. Today, it's a booming haven for ethnic restaurants, high-end boutique shopping and rich people. Our house was a brick-and-board postwar two-story: Three bedrooms, a bath, a one-car garage converted into a den. It occupied a corner lot, with trees and a fenced-in backyard.

A house. My house. Nobody living above us or below us; there were no shared walls or exotic kitchen smells. We had a partly finished basement where we could play our records loud and not disturb anyone except our parents. There was a separate dining room and a yard for a dog. Trees and grass, and the Good Humor truck in June.

And just like that, I had a brother and a sister, too. I was ten years old, not so old I'd become set in my ways. I could welcome a new family, even the instant kind. I'd never come home to an empty house again, and I didn't need a key on a shoestring.

We lived in that house for four years. They were good cocoon seasons. No surprises. I had close friends and sleepovers. I played Little League. I was on a wrestling team. I shared a bedroom with Jeff and a life with everyone. I felt loved and secure in a way I never had before. All these people, they care about me, and they aren't going away.

I still go back to that Bethesda house. Every fall, my work takes me to Baltimore. I rent a car at the airport and point it south, down the Baltimore-Washington Parkway to Interstate 495 to Old Georgetown Road. I park in the old neighborhood, and I walk around, calm with happy yesterdays.

No one else in my family does this. And they think I'm nuts for doing it myself. Jeff still lives within an hour's drive, and he hasn't been back since we moved. No matter.

Can a house inhabit a soul? What business does a brick-

and-board structure have, burrowing into my essence that way? I haven't lived there in more than 40 years and yet the place haunts me like the kindest ghost.

Things were good for me there for the first time. No surprises.

WE BROUGHT JILLIAN HOME from the hospital to her own room. It faced the back of the house and afforded a pretty and pastoral view of the mature woods that rose up almost immediately as the yard ended. The limbs of a 100-year-old shagbark hickory peered into the window. Squirrels occasionally danced there, doing some snooping of their own.

During her pregnancy, Kerry had bought for all our relatives some rolls of plain, white wall border a foot wide, several pints of primary-colored paint and a few dozen empty baby-food jars. She put the paint, the jars and strips of the border in individual boxes, with these instructions:

"Where I marked your name and color, please make a handprint with the paint, and sign it underneath."

Grandmother Daugherty, red. Grandma Jean, blue. Aunt Debra, green. Every relative got a box. The aunts and uncles and grandparents and cousins. Everyone from Hopewell and Aliquippa and every precinct where my family had landed. The Phillipses and the Daughertys, the Coopers and the Allisons. The Turneys and the Ryans. Kerry's sister, Janis, her husband, Marc, and their two sons.

Everyone dipped his hand into a color, and laid it on the border. They all lent our little girl a hand. We brought Jillian home to this room with its border of family hands, its beautiful backyard and its nosy squirrels. Twenty-two years later, it was still her room.

Kerry and I came from different ends of the family ideal. We arrived at the center with one thing in common: Our kids would have the love and stability that ought to be every kid's birthright. A parent on the kitchen floor, bleeding from the wrists, isn't something you're likely to forget. Nor is a childhood spent in the loving idyll of an extended family.

Kerry wanted her kids to have the childhood she had because it was familiar. I wanted that, too, because for me it was anything but.

At various times, Jillian has lacked for things along the "typical" kid continuum: Friends, sleepover invitations, car dates, spring-break trips to the beach. Some of the grand and happy attachments of high school were not meant to be. The daily bone on bone we would encounter was never so strong that it infiltrated our four walls, though. Home was a sanctuary. The place to go when nowhere else mattered, filled with loving hands.

We've lived in the same house for 26 years. That's 22 years longer than I've ever lived anywhere else. It's the only home Jillian and Kelly have ever known. Subconsciously I made a promise to myself, as an eight-year-old twirling that apartment key, that if I ever had kids they would have a life that didn't wobble and a home that didn't scare them.

Kerry shared that, even if she approached it from a far more sylvan path.

I didn't have a dark childhood, only a dark event. My dad

loved me. Elsye rescued me. Jeff and Deb were willing co-conspirators in my personal happiness plot. The scene for my happy ending was the house in Bethesda. The past informs the present. Who we are is owed to where we've been. There is always a footprint.

Every summer, my son, Kelly, and I go to Montreat. We hike Lookout and appreciate the memories we've made and will keep making. I say a silent hello to Mom.

On Jillian's first night of her life at home, she slept in the family room, by a fire we kept stoked all night, in a house with no power. An ice storm had downed the power lines. But the bad weather broke that second day. Sun nudged the clouds. It was warm. Fall had returned. The second night, and every night after that, Jillian slept in the room facing the backyard. Her room. As we laid her down to sleep, a slice of moon brightened the floor of her bedroom, a luminous tribute to a loved child who would avoid the surprises.

CHAPTER 3

Kerry

Jillian will define Jillian.
—KERRY

Bringing Jillian home was not like bringing Kelly home. There was joy, but it was latent. There was hope, but it was trying to get its sea legs. There was determination. That was Kerry's. It was as if God were saying to her, "You want raising children to be your life's work? Well, have I got a job for you."

For nine months, Kerry had prayed for some divine act that would allow her to remain at home with the baby. She had returned to work as a physical education teacher six weeks after Kelly was born. It was wrenching. Teaching school was not Kerry's calling. Motherhood was.

After graduating from Edinboro (Pennsylvania) State College in 1976 with a bachelor of science in Health and Physical Education, she took a job teaching high school PE in West-minster, Maryland, at the time a rural outpost an hour west of

Baltimore. She coached field hockey and gymnastics as well.

Three years later, I graduated from Washington & Lee University with a journalism degree and a job I would start three days after graduation: Beat reporter for a small daily paper, covering the town of Westminster, Maryland. By 1981, I was the sports editor of the daily paper in Westminster. Kerry and I met on the job.

I WAS INTERVIEWING HER after one of her team's games. My last question was, "Do you want to go out sometime?"

Okay, she said and asked when.

I knew I couldn't date someone I had to write about, and I didn't figure she would say yes so I said, "I don't know . . . after your season." I asked her out in October, even though her season had another six weeks to go. She thought I was strange.

We dated for 18 months and got married in April 1983. Kelly arrived in July 1986. In the months before his birth, I'd done the required dad-in-waiting things: Attended couples' Lamaze classes ("Breathe, dear"), constructed baby furniture, even placed a tape recorder of rock-and-roll music on Kerry's stomach so the child would be born with an instant Rolling Stones affection.

I wasn't into it the way Kerry was, though. Maybe it was our age difference. She was 32, I was 28. It could have been that I didn't see the need to complicate the great life we shared. It took me years to appreciate Kelly the way Kerry did from the start. Kelly was born at 7:00 in the morning on July 5, 1986. I covered a baseball game that night.

I'd resisted having another child after him, for many of the same reasons I'd resisted having him. The selfish gene did not recede.

"I want Kelly to have a brother or sister," Kerry said.

"I was an only child for nine years," I replied. "My formative years, right?"

"That explains why you're so antisocial," she said.

She might have had a point. Being an only child means you don't have to fight for the last piece of cake or wear someone's used shirts. You exist in a childhood world of one. Life lessons such as sharing and patience and how to deliver a punch to the shoulder were not daily occurrences in my life. I didn't have to learn to get along.

"I did okay," I suggested lamely.

"Kelly will do better," Kerry replied.

Kerry wanted Kelly to have what she'd had, a sibling with whom he could share a deep relationship. I didn't automatically see the connection. "Just because he has a little brother or sister doesn't mean they'll have a great relationship," I said. My dad and his brother, my uncle Dave, spent half their lives not speaking. I went almost 30 years before reconnecting with another uncle, my birth mother's brother. My cousins and I have next to no relationship. And so on.

My side of the family could be an episode of *Dr. Phil*. On the good days. I was a little jaded on the subject.

I relented, eventually, because relenting is part of a husband's job description, and also because I agreed with Kerry. It would be good for Kelly to have a sibling. And Kerry wasn't getting any younger. She'd be 35 years old by the time the new baby was born.

In the months before Jillian's arrival, Kerry eased Kelly

into the idea of being a big brother. She made him a book, which she called *God Bless the Baby*. In it, a reluctant Kelly says he doesn't want to share his house, or his possessions, with a stranger. Kerry illustrated it by taking pictures of Kelly while he was doing daily Kelly-things. In the story, when the baby arrives, Kelly decides sharing isn't such a bad way to go.

The book was just one example of Kerry's earnestness as a mother. Given my preference for work, we made a decent partnership. The kids-and-careers balance is tough to find. We found it. I wrote. Kerry nurtured.

Kelly had homemade Halloween costumes. For one of them, Kerry had him lie down on the floor, then traced his body on a big sheet of butcher paper so she could make a pattern for a clown outfit. His birthday parties always had a theme—one year it was Robin Hood, the next it was the Teenage Mutant Ninja Turtles.

Her attention was vital because my job required me to be away frequently, covering a Final Four or a Super Bowl or a Kentucky Derby—whatever the calendar dictated. I missed birthdays because I was at the World Series. Father's Day found me at a golf course, covering the U.S. Open. If this is April, it must be the Masters.

Even when I was home, I wasn't always home. The tyranny of a daily column often left me dwelling on today's effort and pondering tomorrow's. Physically, I could be sitting in the family room and we could be having a conversation, but I was really thinking about what I was going to write next.

Kerry could say to me, "Kelly tied his shoes for the first time today," and 30 minutes later I'd ask, "How close is Kelly to tying his shoes?"

It was frustrating for her, not just because she knew I hadn't been paying attention. Kerry knew my work obsessions were denying me precious memories. Firsts are firsts for a reason, she'd say.

That changed when Jillian came, and our lives entered a completely different phase, one we didn't request and never anticipated. Jillian's birth forced us to downshift our lives, to match her pace better. To say we moved forward isn't entirely accurate. Kerry moved forward. I hitched a ride.

"We need a plan," she announced a few days after we left the hospital. "I've cried. I've been upset. I'm done with that. Jillian has Down syndrome. What can we do about it? It's not like we can't help her. She has something we can do something about."

Within weeks after Jillian was born, Kerry had her enrolled in all manner of therapies. Early intervention, the experts called it. Jillian began occupational and physical therapies when she was two months old. Speech therapy followed soon after. She was eventually in a play group with other kids with Down syndrome at Cincinnati Children's Hospital.

At home, she entered the raucous world of a three-year-old boy and a shepherd-collie Kerry had named Deja-Vu. We treated her just as we treated Kelly. We decided there would be no special Down syndrome dispensations. Kelly, who didn't quite grasp the concept, wondered if he could still play with his sister, "even though she has the Down syndrome." We demanded he do so.

We had thought that Kerry would go back to work when the school year started after Jillian was born. That could not happen now. One parent had to be on duty for the job of building the better Jillian. It wasn't going to be me. Work defined me. I couldn't imagine forsaking my career to raise a child. When Jillian arrived, Kerry couldn't imagine anything else.

"What's better than raising a productive human being?" she asked.

My moods and self-worth fluctuated daily, depending on how well I thought my column was going. I was working for the *Cincinnati Post* then, writing four sports columns a week. Getting a column was a plum appointment. The *Post* hired me from New York, where I'd worked as a sports feature writer at *Newsday*, on Long Island.

Most columnists are egotists. A need to be noticed comes with the territory—as does a snobbish belief that we are the best writers at the paper. Without us, there'd be no paper. This isn't true, of course, but some of us need that attitude to do what we do.

Writing a column isn't like covering a beat. You have to know a little about a lot: A mile wide and an inch deep. You have to be connected to those with wisdom about subjects you don't have the authority to speak about. You have to have an edge to your personality, even if that edge is soft. You have to have the stomach to face people you criticize. And you have to be prepared to grind out four columns a week, 50 weeks a year, whether you've got news you can react to or not.

Everyone thinks he can write a sports column. Everyone should try coming up with something to write in February.

The column assumes a tyrannical existence in a columnist's life. In those first few years of figuring out how to do it, the column ruled me. The minute I finished each day's column, it was time to start thinking about tomorrow's. Some days, the words flowed from brain to keyboard, strong and un-impeded. Others, they gathered some place in between, and took the day off. I'd go through stretches of ineffectiveness—writer's clamp—that made me miserable to live with.

"Why Can't I Do This!?" I'd yell to no one. Kerry and Kelly knew not to come into my office during those times. The dog tucked her tail between her legs. "I've been doing this my whole damned life!" I'd wail to the gods. "And now, it just . . . STOPS?" It wasn't unlike a hitter in baseball who runs into a slump. You don't know how you get into it or why you come out of it. Only that when it happens, it drives you mad.

So I was not always a gold-medal dad. I would be standard-issue. I wasn't going to be Gibraltar. Gibraltar was Kerry's department. Raising Kelly was who she was. And Jillian. Jillian would be Kerry's life's work. Any pressure Kerry felt was for Jillian to do well, even to thrive. Kerry assumed total responsi-bility for Jillian's success or failure. She knew she couldn't cure Jillian's Down syndrome. She could help Jillian overcome it.

"I could help her so that she could do everything everyone else could do," Kerry said. "If I didn't do all I could do—the exercises, the therapy, the reading of books to her, practicing her letters—it would be my fault. That was my responsibility."

Kerry was there to keep stitched the fabric of Jillian's prog-ress. While I was out playing in the toy department of the newspaper, she took Jillian to therapies and doctor's appoint-ments and play groups. She immersed herself in the latest news. She became expert in the vital and mundane laws de-signed to give Jillian a chance. She took part in parent forums. Eventually, parent groups invited her to speak.

It's an amazing gift, motherhood. Some use it better than

others. Some have it presented to them in ways they'd never imagined. Kerry made it look easy. Her skill allowed me to pursue my passion.

I look back now, with wonder and with a small sadness at what I missed. Kerry will offer a Remember-When, and I won't remember. It's as if I'm hearing it for the first time. It could have been my way of coping with Jillian's disability, or simply what I thought fatherhood should be. My dad was a rock when I needed him. He didn't feel the need to be highly engaged otherwise. When my brother and I had kids of our own, my dad enjoyed them, but he didn't dote. "I'm not a professional grandparent," he explained.

He could be emotionally vague. I inherited some of that. I earned the money so Kerry could stay home and take care of the children. I wasn't completely disengaged; I just directed my energies differently.

Kerry prepared diligently when she spoke to parent groups and attended school meetings regarding Jillian's education. She'd ask if I wanted to know what she'd learned. I said no. I told her I had confidence in her ability to do everything right. This was true, but it was also an easy cop-out for someone who lacked the special determination to be a full-fledged partner in building the better Jillian.

I attended the meetings. I could make forceful appeals if things didn't go as we believed they should. Beyond that, I was furniture. If Kerry couldn't explain an issue involving our daughter to me in ten words or less, she lost me.

Kerry spent a decade at home, and she never strayed from the mission, giving her full attention to the smallest details. Every toy or game she bought for Jillian had some educational purpose. No mother-daughter conversation was ever frivolous. The books Kerry chose for Jillian were not simpleminded or designed only to entertain. They were educational or award winners. If Kerry could have found a Caldecott-winning alphabet book, she would have bought two copies.

When she was in a hurry, she might have picked up Kelly and carried him upstairs for his nap. But she never picked up Jillian. She wanted Jillian to master the stairs herself. Eventually, that extended to social skills. Kids with Down syndrome are overtly, sometimes overly, affectionate. It's endearing. It also adds to the stereotype. Early on, Kerry had Jillian shaking hands and making eye contact.

She also worried that all the attention paid Jillian would make Kelly feel neglected. Kerry took Kelly to Jillian's therapy sessions. She involved him in Jillian's games. She told him how much she loved him.

In ways subtle and profound, Jillian got something else from Kerry: An iron will she wielded like a magic wand. Jillian would always do what she set out to do.

With Jillian, Kerry got the sibling she wanted for Kelly, but she also got to do the work she'd always wanted to do. How it came about could not have been predicted. Jillian was my daughter. She was Kerry's monument. Construction was just beginning.

CHAPTER 4

Therapy

We never had the luxury of being able to
close our eyes and pretend.
—FRANK DEFORD, FROM *ALEX,*
THE LIFE OF A CHILD

What they don't tell you about having a child with Down syndrome, what they can't possibly know, is that very quickly you develop a syndrome of your own. It is equal parts fear and determination, anguish and love. It produces an alchemy of hope and sadness, a strange human metallurgy that stiffens your spine as your heart cracks. You don't know what to do. So you do everything, and even then, everything isn't enough. But its purpose is to sew you tightly so the worry doesn't win.

We chased information. We kept moving. That way we eased our grief. We knew we couldn't cure Jillian. We also believed it was worth the attempt. We became wrapped up in a measured mania. Not an obsession, just constant motion.

You can't drown in sorrow when you're spending all your time swimming.

We stayed afloat on the hope of the present. What can we do today to make Jillian better? The future became immediately and forever constricted. Our lives became a sports cliché. We took it one play at a time.

We had left the hospital as soon as we could. A nurse had asked Kerry if she wanted to be moved from the maternity ward. "Why would I want to do that?" my wife had asked. "I just had a baby." The implication was that the maternity ward was a happy place. Our presence was anything but. We didn't want to stay anyway. It wasn't a happy place.

The hospital staff had offered mounds of literature. Armies of the well-meaning—doctors, nurses, counselors, volunteers from the local Down syndrome association—provided printed advice. "Here are some things you might like to know," they had said. The pamphlets had titles like, "What Is Down Syndrome?," "Knowing Your Baby" and "Up Syndrome." We thanked them and threw the pamphlets in the trash. The writers knew their subject from a clinical perch; some even had firsthand experience. They did not know Jillian.

Kerry and I had no desire to discover what Jillian wouldn't do. Not that first day, or any day thereafter. We didn't want anyone defining Jillian. We would leave that to her.

"They didn't give us that stuff when Kelly was born," Kerry said. We were insulted and in denial, both. "I just assumed Jillian would do all the things everyone else does," Kerry said. Tell us what she can do.

We developed a few mantras that day. They would expand and evolve, but the resolve they implied never did. The sayings got us through the days. They were a banner that conspired against doubt and pain. We didn't want to know what was behind the curtain. We didn't want to know what was beyond the next five minutes. We plowed ahead, repeating phrases:

All You Can Do Is All You Can Do.

Nothing Is Definite.

Let Jillian Be Jillian.

And, above all: Expect. Don't Accept.

You should get what you expect. Not what you accept. For us, it was the difference between battling and settling, between daydreams and real ones. It is how we've helped Jillian become Jillian. Her limitations are obvious. What's less apparent is how many of those limitations disappear when we expect better and more from her and from ourselves—and from everyone charged, however briefly, with Jillian's progress. Jillian's potential would not be tethered to anyone's preconceptions.

I read something not long ago in a book called *Choosing Naia: A Family's Journey* by Mitchell Zuckoff. In it, a pediatrics professor at the University of Connecticut named Robert Greenstein, who was also director of the Division of Human Genetics at Connecticut Children's Medical Center, is quoted as saying to the couple whose unborn daughter, Naia, had already been diagnosed with Down syndrome: "Nine out of ten things people are going to tell you about Down syndrome are going to be wrong. So it's up to you. If you choose to have this baby, you have to be the expert. Take leadership. People are going to follow your lead. If you're really positive about it, other people will be positive about it."

We too were overloaded with facts and figures in those

early weeks and months. We'd see a geneticist and therapists of all types. Books were recommended and passed along, appointments were made. And we began to realize how different our lives would become.

During Jillian's first few weeks, when people didn't know what to say, what we heard most was, "God doesn't give you anything you can't handle." I didn't know what that meant. If Kerry and I were unfit parents, we wouldn't have had a child with a disability? That seems an incentive to be a lukewarm parent. If God judged us barely adequate at bringing up kids, He wouldn't have determined we were competent enough to raise a daughter with Down syndrome?

Well-intended people had trouble talking about our daughter. The phone kept ringing, and people were surprised when Kerry answered. Why would someone who just had a baby with Down syndrome be answering the phone? "It's like they thought someone had died, and the next of kin doesn't want to come to the phone," Kerry said.

The nicest people said the strangest things. "I'm sorry" sounded both appropriate and offensive. We had no good reaction when someone said that. If we said "thank you" it affirmed that, yes, we were sorry, too. When we weren't.

"How are you?" didn't quite get it, either. That's a common enough question. We got it when Kelly was born. The tone was different with Jillian, though. The question seemed freighted with genuine concern for our emotional well-being.

"We're fine," Kerry and I would say.

"Don't worry, it will be all right" was another well-meaning reaction to Jillian's arrival.

Who says it isn't all right now?

I said "uh-huh" a lot.

"We're so sorry," someone might say.

Uh-huh.

"Will she get better?" was another.

I don't know. Better than what?

She didn't have the flu. "It's not a disease," I told someone. "It's who she is."

Not long after Jillian was born, we had her baptized. A day or two before the event, Kerry mentioned in passing to the minister that Jillian had Down syndrome. "That's all right," he said. "We'll baptize her anyway."

We learned to interpret people's words through the filter of their best intentions. When someone said, "I'm sorry," what that person meant was, "I know you're sad and disappointed now, but it will get better." When someone said, "Will she get better?" they wanted to know if through hard work and determination, Jillian could eventually overcome her disability. Her Down syndrome-ness.

The reactions were a sort of foreshadowing for Kerry and me. So this is how the world is going to be: Hesitant, fearful, well-meaning and removed. It would be filled with people offering condolences.

Less than five weeks after she was born, we enrolled Jillian in physical, occupational and speech therapies. She had checkups that went far beyond the normal baby-doctor visits because babies with Down syndrome come with a giant catalog of potential health sadness: Eye issues, stomach issues, holes in their hearts that have to be closed with surgery.

Other things happened, too. Good things. Life lessons happened daily. We learned that compassion, like charity, can be both selfless and selfish. Doing for others makes us feel good about ourselves. Attending to Jillian's needs was part of my job as her father, of course. But in those first days and weeks of her life, the feel-good I got far exceeded the effort I put in on her behalf. Jillian needed my attention. No more, though, than I needed hers.

"C'mere, Jillie," I'd say.

She couldn't come here yet, not at three weeks. She might lift her head, though, and aim her gaze in my direction. I'd grab her ankles and pull her gently across the rug in the family room. "Time for your massage. People pay good money for this stuff."

Jillian was on her back, staring up at me with perfectly round brown eyes that looked like chocolate chips. She'd started cooing almost as soon as she came home. "A-oooh," she'd say. It was a foreshadowing of words to come. Rivers of words, torrents—not all of them sensible or comprehensible. We would never have to worry about Jillian speaking. Occasionally, we would wish she'd stop.

"Okay, sweets," I'd say. With my thumbs, I'd rub the palms of Jillian's hands and the soles of her feet. The doctors said touching was very important early on; it stimulated the nerves. Also, kids with Down syndrome can have an aversion to touch. They recommended the rubbing to remedy that. I'd have done it anyway. It felt good. I needed that. Therapy for the therapist.

Working her tiny hands and feet came with a peace all its own. My thumb practically covered Jillian's palm. It was maybe a half shoe-size smaller than the sole of her foot. Pressing lightly made Jillian happy. Her eyes assumed an expressive softness. Early on, we understood that Jillian would be what the doctors and textbooks call "cognitively delayed." We also realized at about the same time there would be nothing delayed about her emotions. Jillian could love and be loved.

I've thought about that often over the years. What if Jillian had been born severely autistic? If she had been limited in her ability to show us affection, how much harder would our lives have been? We immediately related to Jillian on a basic human level. Her personality helped us deal with that. We rubbed her hands and feet; she stared back, enthralled. The transaction made all of us happy. We all fell in love. What if that hadn't happened?

Jillian was "floppy" as well. That's a dismissive way of saying she had low muscle tone. The physical therapists attacked that. Our at-home regimen was simply to work Jillian's arms and legs up and down, as if we were maneuvering the appendages of a Barbie doll. Jillian wasn't much bigger than a Barbie doll, so it made sense.

We'd brush her, too. We had a small, soft-bristled brush, the kind you might use in the shower. Three times a day, we brushed Jillian's skin, all over. She liked that. "A-oooh," she said. If I found myself snagged in the weeds of the column and in need of something to take my mind off it, I'd come down from my office in the spare bedroom to do the rubbing and the brushing.

Trying to be topical and entertaining in print four or five days a week isn't always easy. On the days when the words are graceful and the subject compelling, it can be like stealing money. On the other days, it's like putting your brain in a vise. I'd start swinging and missing, and I'd want to kill my laptop. Instead I'd walk downstairs and treat myself to giving Jillian a massage. It might not remove the writer's clamp, but at least I wasn't breaking anything.

FOR ME, MUCH OF what's been written by parents of children with Down syndrome takes on a pitying and self-absorbed tone. What's going to happen to us? Why did this happen to me? This isn't the child I wanted. My Book about My Syndrome.

Guilt is common. Guilt for being older, when the risks are greater for having a child with a disability. Guilt for feeling sad about having a baby not seen as perfect. Guilt for lamenting the child you didn't have, and the remorse you feel because of it.

Kerry and I had no guilt or remorse. We did nothing wrong. A child is born, and she's perfect except she has an extra chromosome. We do what we can, the best we can. We take the situation on our terms. Guilt wasn't in the playbook.

Others who have written on the subject express a need for forgiveness. As if they have brought into the world an unsatisfactory human being.

Kerry and I didn't need forgiveness. We didn't expect it. We didn't have time to think about it. There was no need to "forgive" Jillian for who she was. It would have detracted from who she could become.

That said, when the calamities of the day subsided and the house turned inescapably still, we were sad. We allowed ourselves that. Kerry sometimes cried during her nightly bath, occasionally wondering if our burden would ever feel light. "I don't know if I can care for her" she said one night.

She could, of course. She has, magnificently. But in the

footlights of the moment, sometimes it's hard to dance.

The bond with your child is thicker when she isn't perfect. Everything exaggerates. Senses, awareness, caring. Slights, perceived and real. Your emotions are sensitive to the touch. In those first few weeks and months, we kept moving because we didn't know what would happen if we stopped. Fairly quickly, Kerry and I realized Jillian wasn't the only one who needed therapy.

WE NEEDED SOMETHING BEYOND the perpetual motion and striving. An affirmation, some sort of intimate reassurance that, truly, everything would be all right. For me, it came with a dance.

At the end of each day of that first year, I curled my right forearm beneath Jillian's bottom. The fingers of my left hand cupped the back of her head, which at that point wasn't much bigger than a softball. Her arms hung on my shoulders, like wisteria on a plantation oak. Her head fit like a violin between the top of my shoulder and the base of my jaw. I cued a version of the song "Goodnight, My Love" that Los Lobos had recorded for the soundtrack to the movie *La Bamba*.

"May I have this dance, my lady?" I asked Jillian.

"Ah-oooh."

And off we went. We orbited the small space of the living room, weightless and silent, but for the breathing. I sang to her:

Goodnight, my love;
Pleasant dreams, sleep tonight my love;
May tomorrow be sunny and bright.

Father and daughter, old and frightened, needy and new, living in the moment, dancing around the room. It was the best we could do.

I was looking for something beyond perpetual motion to help me negotiate the days. I spent a few days after Jillian's birth damning God to hell. A week later, I was back in church. It didn't take me long to stop seeing Jillian's birth as a tragic roll of the chromosomal dice and start seeing it as a lifelong love affair. I still required an emotional brace, though. I needed Jillian to tell me everything would be okay. I needed her presence at my own salvation. She would have to help me through.

May tomorrow be sunny and bright.

Infants need that closeness. It simulates the womb they just left. Doctors tell you to keep them wrapped tightly in the days after birth. Blanket or arms—either will do. I preferred arms. Because deep down, this part wasn't about Jillian at all.

If you should awake, in the still of the night
Please, have no fear
I'll be there, you know I care
Please give your love to me.

I didn't *want* to hold Jillian; I *needed* to hold her. My sadness was large. My need to protect against it was overwhelming. So I hugged for dear life, just to feel good about something. If I hugged Jillian hard enough, maybe the Down syndrome would go away. Please give your love to me. At the end of each day, my daughter performed therapy on me. She danced with me, around the room.

All we can do is all we can do. We aren't remarkable, Kerry and I. We lined up the mantras all in a row, like well-trained soldiers, and they did our bidding. Trails will be blazed, moons will be jumped. Jillian will decide who she is, as much as humanly possible. All that will happen, you will see.

First, though, we danced.

I held Jillian in my arms and danced a crescent around the room. The space filled with the light from a starry sky as we circled gently around the days of our lives. What is not possible?

May tomorrow be sunny and bright.

And then she almost died.

CHAPTER 5

Dying to Breathe

If children have the ability to ignore all odds and percentages, then maybe we can all learn from them. When you think about it, what other choice is there but to hope? We have two options, medically and emotionally: Give up, or fight like hell.
—LANCE ARMSTRONG

Jillian was five weeks old when she returned to the hospital, literally dying to breathe.

I can't begin to explain what it is like to see a 6-pound, 15-ounce child diminish before your eyes. Words have not been made to bridge the gap between standard-issue fear and outright terror. We spent the first five weeks of Jillian's life worrying about Down syndrome. Suddenly, Down syndrome was the least of our concerns.

She had been having trouble breathing, which isn't uncommon for babies with Down syndrome. Their lungs are often slow to develop, and their nasal passages are small. We first thought she had a cold that, with help from doctors, wouldn't last too long.

Quickly we realized the problem was that Jillian was not equipped to fight the virus that was creating a mucus that stuck like chewing gum to her impossibly small lungs. The textbook definition of bronchiolitis is "a virus [that] enters your baby's respiratory system and causes the bronchioles, the smallest airways in the lungs, to become swollen and irritated. Mucus collects in the bronchioles and interferes with the flow of air through the lungs."

When a child is deeply ill, the world constricts and becomes a very simple place, settled by fear and defined by the four walls of a hospital room. Life is a narrow tunnel in which there are no choices, no options, no decisions to be made. It's only you, the tunnel and your child.

Jillian lay small in her hospital crib at the center of a nest of tubes. She was hooked up to machines that hydrated her, monitored her heart rate and the level of oxygen in her blood. Tubes ran into her chest and abdomen. She had an oxygen monitor attached to her tiny index finger. It was metal and glowed red. Antibiotics dripped into her body. Wires that were held in place by tiny, circular Band-Aids ran from her chest to a monitor on the wall.

She didn't know what was going on. She had no idea there was a chance that, if she didn't respond to the aerosol treatments and if she kept losing weight, she'd be put on a ventilator, and that could cause brain damage.

We wore masks in the room even though we really didn't

want to. We didn't want Jillian to be scared. When Kelly came to visit his little sister, he remained in the hall, waving at her from the window.

The monitors beeped and buzzed. Aural terror. The machine that measured the oxygen concentration in Jillian's blood was especially horrific. It had a habit of beeping several times an hour, usually after Jillian had shifted in her crib and moved the monitor wires. Each time, a nurse would come in, shut it off and tell us not to worry.

Kerry got the message. After a day or so, she calmly told a nurse that the "stupid oxygen machine" was going off again.

I wasn't able to do that. I couldn't rein in my fear. Every time the oxygen machine beeped, I reacted as if I'd been stabbed. It was the soundtrack of my despair. I wondered if it would ever stop. I began to see the infernal beeping machine as a metaphor for the rest of our lives.

We'd been doing okay, coping. The therapies were starting, Jillian was on a schedule of eating, napping, dancing with me and going to bed. Kelly was in preschool. A calming normalcy had returned. After a few months, we wanted nothing more than for the world to stop spinning so fast.

Kerry kept detailed notes during those first several weeks, handwritten in pencil in a short, spiral notebook. The jottings helped her keep track of what the whir of doctors and therapists were saying. They also slowed down the world. As such, they were therapy, too:

10/31, Weight, 6 pounds, 6 ounces
9:30: Dr. Perez, echocardiogram at Children's Hospital

> *1:00: Dr. DeBlasis, two-week checkup, PKV retest*
> *EKG, Dr. Schwartz. Right side of the heart apparently en-*
> *larged. Sonogram needed, to see if opening between right*
> *and left side has closed. Small hole between chambers*
> *should close by itself. Re-exam in 3 months.*

I took Jillian to the 1:00 p.m. appointment with Dr. Nancy DeBlasis, Jillian's pediatrician. I was armed with Kerry's questions:

Why do there seem to be soft spots all over Jillian's head?

What type of Down syndrome does she have?

Are we feeding her the right amount?

Why does one eye seem to be lazy?

Dr. DeBlasis offered reassurance. She was sure the soft spots would close. Jillian has trisomy 21, the most common form of Down syndrome. Jillian was eating properly. We were told to feed her formula every three hours, four ounces at a time. She should gain one ounce a day. The lazy eye was no cause for alarm.

The doctor noted that Jillian had a small umbilical hernia that should disappear by age five.

She asked that we bring Jillian back in a week, and Kerry's hieroglyphics kept us straight about each appointment.

> *11/7, Dr. DeBlasis: Weight, 6 pounds, 12 ounces*
> *Good muscle tone*
> *Weight gain OK. Check again in two weeks*
> *Put silver nitrate on belly button to cauterize it. (Not com-*
> *pletely closed yet.) Check for any oozing to indicate it's still*
> *not closed.*
> *See back in two weeks.*

We ordered our days around these notes. They were the blueprint for how we'd begin the lifetime task of building the best Jillian. New, enthusiastic parents want to do everything right. The totally dependent life they've created deserves nothing less.

It was the same with Jillian, only more so because of an extra chromosome. We fretted over feedings and naps and having a consistent bedtime. We kept small objects out of the crib, we laid Jillian on her back when it was time for her to sleep. We had the baby monitor on the dresser.

We also worried if her tiny ear canals would ever be clear and if her heart ventricles would close voluntarily, or if surgery would be required. We felt her head for the softness where the skull bone had not yet spread.

Jillian was always congested; her little lungs never welcomed an easy breath. We'd lay her in her crib and listen. Jillian's breaths were a titanic struggle. They sounded like a wind gust rippling a flag. Place a paper bag over your mouth. Breathe in. It makes a racket. That was Jillian, sleeping on her back, in her crib, swaddled in a pink sleeper. A worrisome racket, always wheezing.

> *11/22: Saw Dr. McConville for Jillian's congestion. Mc-Conville said bad cold. Treat with salt water drops and suction out.*
> *Must watch feedings. Jillian lost weight: 7 pounds, 2 ounces.*

We did as we were told. We put the saline drops in Jillian's nose. She wailed. We would take a plastic suction device, nearly a foot long, that was narrow but for the rubber bulb at one end, and we'd squeeze the bulb, then gently put the narrow plastic end into each nostril, before releasing the bulb. Jillian wailed. She made such a fuss we thought the world was ending. The little girl who couldn't wait to be born had no trouble expressing her feelings after she'd arrived. Squeeze and release. Squeeze and release. Wail and wail.

> *11/23: Thanksgiving Day. Still congested. Eating less. Began spitting up feedings in early evening.*
> *11/24: Saw Dr. Jones, 4:30, for congestion. Not eating. Vomiting. Weight, 6 pounds, 15 ounces.*

We took Jillian to Children's Hospital that night, and they took a chest X-ray. They hooked her to an IV to give her nutrients and to prevent dehydration. They said she needed aerosol treatments to open her airways. And they said she needed oxygen.

The last item dried my throat. Needed oxygen? I didn't know what that meant, except it couldn't be good. My daughter couldn't breathe on her own. I knew she wasn't eating, and she was losing weight, but now she couldn't breathe. The simplest acts of survival were suddenly complex. Kerry's careful journaling was becoming a diary of terror. Into the tunnel we went.

> *Had a rough night of it. Seen by Dr. Strait. Believed to be bronchiolitis, X-rays tomorrow should confirm.*

THE X-RAY CONFIRMED THE diagnosis, sending us into ten days of purgatory.

Jillian was admitted into isolation. Doctors couldn't risk her incurring any additional infections. They placed her in a crib. Several times a day, doctors moved her into a tent in her crib and gave her aerosol treatments designed to open her airways and give her lungs some relief. After the aerosol, they suctioned, same as we did at home. Jillian wailed for them too.

Then we tried to get a few ounces of formula into our sick, angry child.

> *11/26, 1 a.m.: Aerosol treatments ordered for every two hours.*
> *3:20 a.m.: Aerosol treatment*
> *5 a.m.: Aerosol treatment*
> *7 a.m.: Aerosol treatment*
> *8:30 a.m.: Aerosol treatment*
> *9 a.m.: Took 1 ounce of formula*

And so on. Aerosol, suction, wailing. Sleep. Formula. Repeat.

> *11/27, 9 a.m.: Dr. Strait came in and said probably three or four more days.*

THREE OR FOUR DAYS of treating and watching for improvement, and Jillian could go home. It wasn't, though. It wasn't three or four more days, which would have been bad enough. That would have meant Jillian was in the hospital for a week or more.

When she couldn't breathe, even with the aid of a tube running into her nose, the nurses put Jillian into what we called "the oxygen box," where she could take in the pumped-in air through her mouth.

The nurses spent a lot of time trying to find places for IVs on Jillian's body. They'd try an arm, and Jillian would pull out the IV, or a vein would collapse. They tried her foot, they tried her head.

"Vein not working," Kerry wrote in the notebook on November 28. *"Must find new one."*

We fed Jillian with a syringe, a specific amount of cc's. Most babies take a 4-ounce bottle. Our baby took 25 cc's. From a syringe.

At 2:15 p.m. on November 28, four days after Jillian had been admitted and three days after the aerosol remedy had been unleashed, a doctor came to Jillian's room and said the wheezing was still obvious and the aerosol treatments had not been effective.

The number of hospital people coming around increased, and the chief resident talked about putting Jillian in intensive care. Two cardiologists studied her and determined that the treatment she was undergoing wouldn't affect her heart, even though the hole hadn't closed completely. Another doctor told Kerry she could feed Jillian, but she had to be careful that Jillian didn't choke on the formula.

At 8:15 p.m., one of the nurses found a worthy vein in Jillian's arm and started a line of something called theophylline to treat the wheezing.

I wondered how much more I could take. I was done watching my daughter get jabbed and punctured and aerosoled. I had had enough of listening to the oxygen monitor and observing the pinched, grave faces of doctors and the patronizing half smiles of the well-meaning nurses. There is no joy in a hospital room—only white knuckles. Jillian's room had acquired an air of patient desperation: *We're going to keep trying things. We hope they will work. But at a certain point, we'll have to consider more extreme options.*

I wondered where all the mercy was in the world—and why none of it had been visited upon my little girl.

Meantime, another doctor arrived to tell us that among the possible side effects of the drug contained in the aerosol were bacterial pneumonia, apnea, hypotension, conjunctivitis. And there was also ventilator dependence. Some doctor or another had mentioned the possibility of brain damage should Jillian become ventilator dependent.

> *11/30, 5 a.m. Tried to feed her. She wasn't interested.*
> *5:45 a.m. Dr. Strait said her wheezing was a little worse.*

With each piece of bad news, each beep of an overactive monitor, each vision of what might happen if things didn't improve, a bit of me took flight. I thought, a man can die without ever leaving the earth. Spiritually, in increments. Each night, I'd leave the hospital in a nether state of disbelief and sadness. In times such as that, you really do say, "This is all a dream, and I am going to wake up a more generous man, grateful for the everyday glory of what I have."

Only this wasn't a dream—so we trudged through the bright, antiseptic halls of Children's Hospital, its walls decorated with crayon pictures of happy kids and their happy families. We'd go home and fall into a brittle sleep, exhausted to our bones, too exhausted to feel. Then we'd do it all again the next day.

Kerry was better about it. She achieved a sort of compromised peace by taking voracious notes. She wrote down the times when she fed Jillian, when Jillian took an aerosol treatment, when her blood was drawn and when another IV was inserted. Kerry took down the names of all the drugs Jillian got, every doctor who visited, and what they said. This kept her occupied and made her feel useful. It also kept the doctors informed and on task.

Sometime around our sixth day into this purgatory trip, Kerry's stoicism snapped. Two bad experiences caused her to lose her composure. The first occurred when nurses tried to give Jillian the wrong medicine. Kerry had asked all of the nurses and doctors to tell her what each medication was, what it was for and how often it was used. As a result, she was pretty knowledgeable about what Jillian was being treated with. Then on this day, Kerry saw a nurse attach to the IV line something not on the list in the notebook.

"She doesn't get that," Kerry said.

"Yes, Mrs. Daugherty, she does. Don't worry," the nurse said.

Kerry insisted a doctor be summoned. She wasn't polite about it. She was also correct. Medicines had been mixed up. A few days later, Jillian was crying uncontrollably in the middle of the day. Crying was bad, if only because it produced mucus in the nose, which drained to Jillian's lungs.

"She's crying because she's hungry. I'll feed her," Kerry said.

"Not now," she was told. "We don't want any liquid in her throat when she's crying."

"She's crying because she's hungry," Kerry insisted. "I know my child."

Again, no.

"Why won't you listen to me?" Kerry yelled, a week of frustration and worry purged in one primal scream.

They listened. Kerry fed Jillian, and Jillian stopped crying.

Still, Jillian was losing weight, and her lungs were not clearing. She'd been in the hospital for a week. We needed something good to happen, and we needed it fast. "I'm starting to get scared" was what I told Kerry. "It's beyond the normal worry."

We were beyond tired. We wore our fatigue like a second skin. It defined us, it was almost a painkiller. By Day 8, we were numb. The hospital ceased being a place of hope. It was a repository for dirges, featuring precise, beeping-monitor solos. We hadn't given up on hope, but we really wanted to see some.

Then suddenly the monitor went off, and the platoon of nurses marched in. I scanned their faces. Nothing. Then one nurse left quickly. Seconds later, two doctors came in.

"What's wrong?" I asked. Kerry and I were told to step back.

We backed up—away from the doctors and the nurses and the crib holding our daughter. Seven people were surrounding the crib. I thought Jillian was going to die. I didn't blame the doctors, the hospital, Kerry or myself then. I didn't blame anyone. I was all out of blame.

Instead, I closed my eyes and prayed this:

"God, do not bring Jillian this far, only to let her leave. You blessed us with her. Let her life be a blessing. She is here for a reason. Her life is not an accident. Do not take her before we find out what that reason is."

Our tight world turned inward another notch: Crib, doctors, Jillian. There was nothing else on the planet, absolutely nothing.

A nurse moved away from the crowd around the crib and left the room. She returned with yet another long needle at the end of yet another long tube. For this latest attempt at finding a suitable vein, the nurses shaved Jillian's head. Kerry, ever the calm portion of this marital unit, approached the crib, sidled between the nurses and collected Jillian's freshly shorn locks. Daughter on the brink, mother collecting hair.

"First haircut," she explained later. "I had to save her hair. The first haircut is the first haircut, no matter where you have it."

Another nurse removed the needle from its sterile packaging, and Kerry knew she was needed there to hold Jillian down before the nurse jammed the needle into the top of my daughter's head. I had to leave the room.

AND THEN THE DAMNEDEST thing happened.

It was odd, it was lucky. It was Jillian being Jillian at the most perfect time, when nothing else would do.

At the feel of the needle, Jillian started screaming down to the tip of her toes. She screamed at the pain of it all and maybe the injustice, too. Jillian might have lacked the smarts to understand what was happening, and the capacity to wonder why it was happening to her. But she knew she was hurting; and she knew she was angry and had had enough. She was done with all of it. She was born on the day of the San Francisco earthquake, and now she was moving her own personal fault line. She was shaking her metaphorical fist.

What happened next is easily described but not easily explained. You could say the force of Jillian's protest shook heaven and earth and, not coincidentally, a great gob of the junk currently fouling her lungs. You could say that Jillian literally screamed the snot out of herself.

It was Jillian saying, "I'm sick of this, and I'm not going to take it anymore." It was a wail that topped all those that came before it, in emphasis, volume and sheer anger. It was like nothing I've ever heard.

THAT TOXIC GOB OF evil mucus dislodged itself from Jillian's lungs and made its way up her throat and out the front door of her mouth. This six-pound child's screaming revolt had achieved what a week's worth of aerosols and meds had not.

I believe that Jillian's spirit saved her life. It saved her for us. She was not going to leave so soon. Too much to do. Too much Jillian to spread around. Much more time required. No time for any more of this hospital.

12/2, 12:30 p.m.: Dr. Jonas, new doctor on rounds. Says Jillian is doing better. Her lungs sound very clear.

The aerosol treatments continued. The suction and the wailing, the feedings, 25 cc's at a time. But now Jillian was doing better. Two days later, they removed the oxygen box from the crib. The day after that, she stopped needing the aerosol. The next morning, we bathed her. And we weighed her. She was 6 pounds, 14 ounces—one ounce lighter than when she'd arrived at Children's Hospital. Only three ounces more than when she was born, six weeks earlier.

There was a knowing in her eyes though. You see it all the time in hospitalized kids. They always appear older than they are, as if the struggling they did with something beyond their control had informed them about life's vagaries in a way that healthy kids will never know.

Sick kids have struggled, they've endured. They own something most of us never will: A wisdom, a patience, an ability to cope. Whatever it is, it belongs to Jillian, and has for 24 years.

> *12/2, 5:30 p.m.: Dr. Brokaw decided to have her stay overnight with no aerosol treatments, to observe, then send her home tomorrow a.m.*

Jillian attacked life from the day she became a member. Jillian has never been less than fearless and engaged. In baseball parlance, Jillian gets her hacks.

There is that. And this:

Her existence has a point. Jillian might have gotten a bad dice roll, but her presence is not happenstance. She is here for something. This is what I took with me from Children's Hospital after 12 days. Jillian survived. She is here for something.

This is what I believed then. This is what I hold dear.

Kerry's last note:

> *12/6: Jillian began cooing at us, and also in response to us.*

Ah-oooh.

CHAPTER 6

Kelly

. . . . and remember to be kind.
—JACKSON BROWNE

The first time Jillian laughed was after Kelly made a face. He'd been working on it for days. He'd contort his gaze into all manner of goofiness.

He would test the elasticity of his nose, up and down and side to side.

"Hey, Jillian, look at me! Look, Jillian!"

He'd use his fingers to pry open his mouth. He'd do fantastic things with his face and tongue. The human gaze is a marvelous instrument of expression. Kelly turned his into Comedy Central. Kelly did this because that's what little kids do, but also even at age three, he was beginning to understand there was something different about his sister.

The first laugh happened when Jillian was two months old and freshly freed from the hospital. What we heard was a staccato rumble from somewhere deep. Kelly was busy making his funny faces, and Jillian was sitting up, propped by the couch.

"Did you hear that?" Kerry said.

I did.

A laugh doesn't seem like much, but we hadn't done a lot of laughing in those first eight weeks. During Jillian's hospital stay, laughter was an obscene, awful foreign language. We had to learn it all over again, and to be grateful for its presence.

It wasn't difficult. We hadn't lost Jillian, and in the process, we'd found something. Calling it "perspective" is clichéd. Everyone who knows someone with a disability talks about the perspective they've gained from the knowing. You might find "perspective" when Jillian is right in front of you. You lose it the next time you're sitting in traffic.

And yet from the moment we left the hospital with Jillian for a second time, we knew nothing would be quite the same. We would not be so busy with each day that we would presume its best moments.

Jillian wasn't struck with our sober single-mindedness. She had no idea. When Kelly was making faces, all Jillian knew was that her brother was making her happy. So she laughed. This was the start of something big.

Eventually, the village embracing and protecting Jillian would spread. As she ventured deeper into the world, her influence would spread, too. At this moment, the village was tight but no less important.

There is no predicting how a kid will react to having a competitor in the house, especially when the new sister has a disability that requires extra attention. But Kelly's eagerness to make his sister laugh was a clear and pleasant beginning and a start toward good things.

We enjoyed the moment. We allowed that. It was extraordinary.

Meantime, Kerry and I worried about how all this attention paid to Jillian would affect Kelly.

He was three years old then and was shy around strangers, but there was nothing strange about his house. He'd called dibs on that from the first. Now, a stranger had arrived and . . . stayed.

Kelly celebrated Jillian's original homecoming by hanging from the mantel in the family room. Jillian was two days old. Kelly had been around three years. He'd earned his spot in the family hierarchy. *She was coming here? To my place? Well, okay. But she can't do what I can do. She can't hang from the mantel.*

His size-two feet dangled a foot above the floor. His fingers were bone-white from clutching the wood. He was incredibly proud of himself. "Look at me!" Kelly announced. "Look at what I'm doing! Jillian can't do this!"

Kelly also told us he had teeth. He did have a full set of gleaming baby teeth, all in a row. "Look at me eat these Oreos! Jillian can't eat Oreos!" Kelly proudly jammed a few fingers into his sister's mouth to advance his theory. "See? No teeth! Jillian can't eat Oreos! Jillian doesn't have teeth!"

Kerry wanted Kelly to have Jillian. She wanted him to have the experience she had with her older sister. Kerry and Janis weren't always best friends. But they were close even when they were apart, in a way only sisters can be. Soon after Jillian's diagnosis was made, nurses at the hospital asked Kerry her most immediate concern.

"I'm worried about my son," she said.

We had named Jillian long before she was born so Kelly could know her before she arrived. We kept him informed of her progress. We didn't want him to feel left out. Kelly felt Jillian kick in the womb. He heard the whoosh-whooshing her heart sounds made on the ultrasound. He watched the video from that procedure. We had a sno-globe that played the Tony Bennett standard "I Left My Heart in San Francisco." Kelly liked to wind it up and put it on Kerry's stomach.

He was ready for a sibling, as much as any three-year-old could be. But maybe not for this sibling.

"Look how much I grew!" Kelly said as he threatened to separate the mantel from the wall.

"We saw you yesterday," I reminded him.

He insisted on tossing a ball in the house. It nearly went through a window. He whooshed like a big wind. "Look at me! I'm fast!" I'm thinking, *So this is how it's gonna be. One kid won't do enough. The other will do too much.*

Their lives began entirely differently. Jillian entered center stage, shouting triumphantly, seeking applause in the footlights. Three years and a few months earlier, her brother had emerged in silence. He was awestruck and simply stared.

Kerry's legs were still airborne, in the stirrups. A doctor stood at the foot of the bed. Beneath his feet lay a wastebasket. I remember thinking, *Is that in case Kelly slides out so quickly, the doctor doesn't catch him?* Headfirst, into a trash can. What a way to begin life.

That didn't happen. Kelly's head emerged first, facedown.

He cork-screwed as he left Kerry's womb, so when he finally arrived, he was looking up at the ceiling. It took him a few minutes to decide he really wanted to be here.

More than two decades later, Kelly is still inquisitive and curious, wary and contemplative. One toe in the water, nine high and dry. He's still checking it all out.

In those first few days after Jillian was born, when we grieved a sad dizziness, we also worried for Kelly. What sort of prologue would all the prenatal introductions provide? Would Kelly love his little sister, or resent her?

That first day home, we paused from watching Kelly's indoor Olympics long enough to eat some lunch. As we ate, it got quiet—not a normal condition in a house with two kids under the age of four.

"What happened?" Kerry asked.

Kerry's dad, Sid, had built Jillian a cradle. Hardwood, with what looked like sled runners on the bottom, so the cradle would rock. Jillian lay in it now, sleeping. Kerry and I went to investigate. Where is Kelly?

He was inside the cradle, curled up beside Jillian, an arm around her waist.

"That's when I knew this would not be an ordinary sibling relationship," Kerry said.

Luckily, it was a big cradle, with enough room for a 6-pound baby and her 40-pound brother. They lay face to face, eyes closed, like nesting dolls.

This is going to work, I thought. *This isn't going to be so bad.*

Kelly started right in with Jillian, helping with her physical therapy. He'd rub the soles of her feet. He'd gently work her arms, up and down and in and out. He'd sit on the floor of the family room and roll a ball to her to improve her hand-eye coordination. He did everything with her that Kerry and I did.

We wanted him to feel needed. It's a great thing for a three-year-old to be needed. Even at that age, when all that matters to you is what matters to you, Kelly learned that his universe contained other stars. "Without Jillian, I would be an entirely different person," Kelly said not long ago.

Less giving, he said. Less understanding, less compassionate. Less aware of peoples' differences and the possibilities they present. Kelly is fortified with a willingness to look outward. "Jillian pushes me to do what I do," he said.

He's 28 years old now. The quiet, observant child has become a man on the cusp. He lives in Brooklyn, New York, where he works at a publishing house. As he once noted to me, seriously but without malice, "I don't want to be a newspaper guy, Dad. I want to be a real writer." Kelly's emergence into adulthood has looked a lot like the day he was born.

He knows things his peers do not. Some of it is innate; Kelly thinks about things. Some came from that six-pound girl, lying next to him in the homemade cradle. Jillian has modeled her behavior after Kelly. Kelly has ordered his life around the lessons Jillian's life has suggested. Things that make the world move: Patience, tolerance, optimism, kindness.

When Kelly was in nursery school, he took Jillian to show-and-tell. "This is my little sister. She has Down syndrome." They'd play for hours in the finished basement. Kelly called it the K and J Club. Jillian's first word was "Kelly." Life was never so fast that Kelly couldn't linger a while for his sister. She was both the tug on his shirt and the push on his aspirations. She

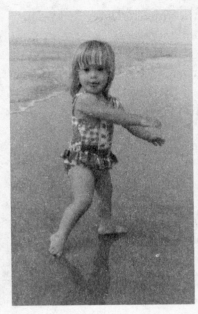

Jillian, age four, on the beach at St. Simons Island, Georgia.

taught him. This is what I thought. I wondered if he felt the same.

He did. He described her as a palm in his back, gently pushing.

For a family, the extra attention paid to a child with a disability is both a strain and a chance. The hours and frustrations march side by side with the little wins and the big lessons. It's hard to know where one stops and the other begins.

Jillian has been the palm in Kelly's back, gently pushing him to read one more chapter of Faulkner before calling it a night. Refine a few paragraphs in that graduate school thesis. Set the alarm 30 minutes earlier. Be glad about it.

Kelly is a deep thinker. He's not good at articulating his thoughts. Jillian gives him a feeling, he says. "Her enthusiasm for life has made me more enthusiastic."

When Kelly was in high school, he'd pile into a borrowed car with his guy friends, and head out on weekend nights to commit high school–guy things. Our common drive is shared with three other families. It's a few hundred yards long. Near its end is a large rock.

When Jillian knew Kelly was going out, she'd walk down

to the rock, sit down and wait for him to leave. Kerry and I watched this scene at least a hundred times:

Kelly would tell us goodnight for the evening and hop in a friend's backseat. They'd cruise down our lane, toward the main road. Just a bunch of high school boys, armed with bravado, itched by insecurities that only cool popularity could scratch. Before they reached the end of the driveway, just before the road, we'd see the red brake light. The car would stop.

Kelly would be awkwardly shoving himself out of what always seemed to be a two-door car. He'd take a few steps, to the rock. He would kiss his little sister on top of her head. We asked him once why he did this and he couldn't ever actually explain it. He just felt it.

We never knew what Kelly's buddies thought about this, or how they felt in the presence of a child with a disability, maybe the first such child they'd ever met. We never asked. We never asked Kelly what caused him to test the cocoon of guy-ness this way. The answer could never be as important as the gesture itself, offered by a teenaged boy deep in the throes of an adolescent's need to conform and belong.

Jillian would walk up the drive after that, smiling. "Kelly kissed me," she'd say.

Kelly made Jillian laugh, in the scary, hopeful days after she left the hospital, when laughter was a salve. His kiss made her smile.

We all smiled about that. We also remembered not to forget it.

CHAPTER 7

The First Angel

Speak in a loud voice, clearly and without fear.
—JONATHAN SPENCE

Jillian was never our child with a disability; she was simply our child. That's how we saw it, but it didn't mean we could make the rest of her world see her the way we did. That required co-conspirators. They had to share our plan for Jillian, which had little room for compromise. They had to come armed with a generous worldview. They had to believe people are only as good as the way they treat each other.

No one is going to think your child is as wonderful as you think she is. What we wanted was a core of people who would look at Jillian and see potential. We needed like minds with loud voices, speaking clearly and without fear.

We needed people like Martha Coen-Cummings, Jillian's speech therapist and first guardian angel. Martha had worked as a speech pathologist for more than a decade when she met three-year-old Jillian Daugherty. "Marfa" taught with compassion, patience and curiosity. She operated from a base of acceptance. She'd been raised that way.

Her father grew up in Seoul, South Korea, the son of American missionaries. He met Martha's mother in Illinois after World War II. The family settled in Highland Park, a well-off, multiethnic suburb on Chicago's North Shore. Martha was the only child on the block who was born in the United States. She was the only one to speak English exclusively; her friends spoke two or three languages. Her father's closest friends were Asian. Martha was as proficient with chopsticks as with a fork.

When Martha visited her friends' homes, she was forever mindful of the cultural mores. Some asked that she remove her shoes at their front door. Others frowned on expressions of affection; no hugging. In one friend's house, Martha was careful not to compliment something unless she was prepared to take the object home with her. Diversity and acceptance were not the norm in 1960s America. They were in Highland Park.

This was the sort of person we needed to help us in the building of a better Jillian.

By the time Jillian and Marfa began what would be a decade-long collaboration, Jillian had been speaking for at least a year. It didn't matter that neither Kerry nor I knew what she was saying.

Listening to Jillian was like stumbling into a lost Amazonian tribe. She was multisyllabic and entirely conversational. Jillian had a lot going on, even if it was foreign to everyone but her. We worried at first that our daughter's disability would deter her willingness to speak. Soon enough, we wondered when she would stop.

At this age, kids begin forming semblances of words. Kelly said "Day-day" when he talked about our dog at the time, Deja-Vu. He said "moash" when he wanted milk. We understood him, occasionally. For Jillian, the "ah-oohs" had given way to more sophisticated pronouncements. They were gibberish, but they were Jillian's unique brand of gibberish, complete with pauses, inflections and exclamation points. Jillian's need to be heard was obvious. Her ability to mix pitches and to vary tones suggested a feeling behind what she was saying. She didn't know the word "happy." But she knew what being happy was.

We would stand in the upstairs hallway, ears pressed to Jillian's bedroom door, eavesdropping on Jillian's filibusters, which were her purest form of expression. Her tones, inflections and occasional laughs and cries showed she was capable of creating her own parallel world, complete with all the standard emotions. They indicated intelligence because smarts are required to invent the friends she employed as partners in the dialog.

And yet, as I listened to my two-year-old, I wondered what transpired in the wide-open spaces between Jillian's brain and her lips. Where did her abundant thoughts go? Did they emerge lucid from her brain's transmitters, pinball around and disappear? Was there some great holding tank for all the thoughts she couldn't articulate?

I pictured a dead-letter office. A lost and found, for the permanently lost.

Jillian had no such worries. She just liked to talk.

Whenever we made the five-hour car trek to Kerry's parents in Pittsburgh, we discovered we could keep Jillian happy simply by giving her a pair of socks. She would pull them on like mittens, then manipulate them with her hands, like puppets. And she would converse with them for five hours straight. Jillian was fluent in her Language For One. Occasionally, she wouldn't even need socks. Popsicle sticks, one in each hand, were suitable for a lengthy chat.

"How can you stand this?" Kerry's sister, Janis, asked at one point.

"Stand what?" Kerry answered.

When Kerry went to Target or Walmart, she'd plop Jillian in a shopping cart, then find her a dress on a hanger. Jillian would pretend the dress was a friend. She and the dress/friend would converse while Kerry shopped in peace.

In the early years of *Saturday Night Live,* the late Gilda Radner performed a solo skit in which she played a teenaged girl, on the four-poster bed in her room, acting out lavish adventures in private. Radner called it "The Judy Miller Show." That was Jillian. She starred in her own, one-woman show, way off Broadway. The Jillian Daugherty Show. These are the times we'd listen in the hall.

As she got older and the words started happening, Jillian would consult with herself: "What do now?" She'd argue with herself: "No way can do that!" She'd console herself: "It OK, Jiwwian."

Even as I marveled at the sounds behind the door, I was sad they weren't finding a home. There was no audience. This most audacious child, who fought to be born and screamed to stay alive: Would she ever have a voice?

We make admirable accommodation for the physically disabled. They park in the close-up spaces. Building codes must include them. Science enables them. A physically disabled president lifted us from a Depression and guided us through a world war. A sprinter without legs competes in the Olympics, on appendages of carbon fiber. The physically impaired negotiate our society with few stigmas attached.

What of those whose speech is limited? Who are we if we can't communicate? How does Jillian embrace the future if she can't articulate it? Without the sky of language, the words can't fly. Listening at her door, we could tell that so much thinking was occurring inside Jillian's head. Would enough of it emerge, recognizable?

Jillian was faithful about attending all of her therapies—physical, occupational and speech—but we knew the speech mattered most. It was important for Jillian to hold a fork or possibly ride a bike, but being able to communicate was vital. It was everything. She met with Martha for an hour each week. Jillian's strength came as much from her character as her intelligence. Want-to overcame IQ. She came ready to learn. She tried anything.

Jillian also wanted to be in control. Martha would offer her choices of books or games. "Clearly, she wanted to be driving my behavior," Martha said.

"No dat," Jillian might say, when faced with a choice of a game or book. "Dis one."

Jillian was slow to learn nuances. She knew what a cat was; she also knew a kitten was a baby cat. She could see their differences. Emotions are more subtle. "What's the difference between glad and happy and joyous?" Martha would ask.

"I'm happy," Jillian would say.

"Are you glad?" Martha would respond.

"No."

"Can you be happy without being glad?"

"No."

"So, you're happy and glad," Martha asked.

"Yes, I am."

"I am joyous when I open my mail," Martha said. "Does that make sense?"

"Yes."

"No, it doesn't," Martha said.

"No, it doesn't," Jillian repeated

"I am joyous when I open my mail, and there is a check in the envelope," Martha corrected.

Semantics matter because speech is nuanced. Just knowing the words, how to pronounce them and what they mean is not enough. If you miss on the nuance and the semantics, even slightly, the meaning is lost.

Jillian also got hung up on pronouns. Instead of saying, "She is going to the store," Jillian might offer, "Her is going to the store." Lots of kids talk that way; most aren't doing it when they're ten years old.

"Me got a new book today," Jillian might say.

"Who? Me?" Martha might reply, pointing at herself. This would throw Jillian. "No. Me," she'd say. "Jillian."

Martha would tell her she meant, "I got a new book today."

Getting the pronouns right would help eliminate what Martha called "baby talk," which would have a big impact on Jillian socially. "She never lacked confidence. She always wanted to express herself. I just had to refine that," Martha said. Much of Martha's work with Jillian came down to memorizing: Verb tenses, for example. I am drinking today. Yesterday, I drank. Tomorrow, I will drink. This was simple, basic stuff, but with Jillian, the learning took longer. The memorization came more slowly and required more repetition. It wasn't unlike a typical child learning a second language.

"Down kids know the words they want to use. As their vocabulary grows, and they introduce multisyllabic words, the articulation issue gets bigger," Martha said.

In later years, as Jillian entered fourth and fifth grades, it wasn't her physical shortcomings that defined and limited her. Jillian never missed a kickball game. Her delayed speech created the growing divide between her and her classmates. Kids picked up on it. They went from trying to understand Jillian—"What did she say?"—to avoiding her.

It didn't help that by the time she arrived in elementary school, the physical characteristics typical of children with Down had become apparent. People who didn't stare before, stared now. Jillian's face was cherubic and smiling—and also a little too round. Her eyes were shaped like almonds, owing to what the doctors label "epicanthal folds." Jillian's nose was obviously flatter than Kelly's. She had small ears and a small mouth. Her teeth were irregular, with lots of space between them. She would need braces. Her eyesight wasn't great, and soon enough she would wear glasses.

She tended to leave her tongue outside her mouth. This, too, is a Down syndrome giveaway. "Put your tongue away," we told her.

Jillian's hands were small, her fingers stubby. She walked in a forward-leaning way, head out front, which is typical of people with Down.

We are an appearance-crazed society. As Billy Crystal noted frequently, while playing a character based on Fernando

Lamas, "Eez better to look good than to feel good." No one judged Jillian at age two by the way she looked. Her Down characteristics were not yet obvious. But that day would come. When it did, we wanted her to be armed with the proper retort. We wanted her to speak clearly enough to say to everyone who stared, "Don't look at me and judge who I am. See what I can become." This was the hope. Its beginning and end was language.

"We're going to see Martha today," we'd declare. And Jillian would respond, "I go to my talk class." Jillian and Martha would work together for almost ten years, an hour a week, playing, reading, sewing the stitches in a tapestry of expression. Martha helped give Jillian a voice.

Achievements aren't instant. Arriving at them is never a straight path. But they do occur. "What you need is to be happy with the small step," Martha said. "All professions need that, but they don't all embrace it. Everything builds."

Families need it too. The small steps sustained us.

Jillian always had desire on her side. She wouldn't have been so verbal if she hadn't been so eager to test the world. Jillian wanted you to know Jillian. Martha gave Jillian her greatest gift. An angel had poured the cement of language into Jillian's foundation. Martha was the first angel.

In the next few years, there would be more, in rapid fire.

CHAPTER 8

Jillian

You want a piece of me?
—JILLIAN

Jillian might have seemed like one of those regimented super-kids who spend their entire lives in the car, heading for this therapy or that class. And we might have come off as those over-engaged parents you try to avoid at parties so you don't have to hear tales of their children's collective awesomeness. We weren't those parents, and we didn't overdo it. Kids need to be kids, most of all. They need time to lie on their backs in the cool summer grass, to just stare at the sky. They need time to do nothing, time to be bored. Boredom is healthy. It encourages creativity. We left Jillian to her own devices lots of the time. The curtain lifted daily on the Jillian Daugherty Show. Only the venues changed.

Jillian was hell-bent on seizing days. She grabbed life the way a knife grabs a filet. Her outlook affected everything she did, from riding a two-wheeler to learning to spell. The best the rest of us could do was keep her in the middle of the road.

We encouraged her independence in all things. Well, most things. When your child is eight or nine years old and seeks wings, you give in by degrees. The training wheels come off, the boundaries are flexed. Life in the front yard becomes a memory. The front yard is for little kids. Big kids go out and discover the world.

Jillian had determined she would be big. And mobile. The girls who lived next door were mobile. One of them was Jillian's age; the other two were younger. They were able to launch themselves up and down the driveway on Cozy Coupes and rollerblades, tricycles, bicycles, even a little electric car. Jillian definitely noticed when they went beyond the shelter of the drive to the neighborhood pool or to chase the bell-chime sounds of the ice cream truck.

Kelly was also mobile. He'd slip the earthly bonds of the house and yard, hop on his two-wheeler and vanish for hours. Jillian believed she was Kelly. On those first few days after school let out, she'd see him leave the house and her face would scrunch into a Jillian-mix of sadness and determination.

"I wanna go," Jillian announced. "My turn."

But she knew her rules were different. We wanted her to be as typical as any kid, but we had to be realistic. For Jillian to be outside, Kerry or I had to be outside—or at least be able to see her from the window. We limited her kingdom to the house and the yard. It was a small kingdom. We wanted her to be free, but we didn't want to see her face on a milk carton.

We were thrilled with Jillian's sociability and fearlessness, but it made for an inspiring and problematic challenge. Our ultimate goal was her independence. We wanted Jillian to test boundaries, take chances. We wanted her to get lost, but we also wanted to be sure she was able to find herself.

How we balanced that act would be the question.

"I wanna go too," she insisted.

"I have a job for you," Kerry said.

"I made my bed, Mom," Jillian answered.

"I need you to deliver these fliers."

"Fli-ers?"

"These invitations to the neighbors," Kerry said.

Kerry belonged to a neighborhood Bunco group. Bunco is a mindless game played with dice. That is all I know about Bunco. Bunco Night was an excuse for the wives to get together, get happy and gossip. It was Kerry's turn to host, and she gave Jillian three fliers: For the Rutkouskys next door and for the Snyders and the Warzalas nearby.

"Yay!" Jillian said.

An irony of life is that it goes too slowly when we want it to go fast, and it goes too quickly when we wish it would slow down. Years aren't really longer when you're 8 years old than they are when you're 68; they just seem that way. Kids are in a hurry. When they're 15, they want to be 16 so they can drive. When they're 20, they want to be 21 so they can drink.

When they're in high school, they want to be out, either to college or a job. When they're in college, they want to graduate. And so on. They push hard on their days. They stretch and test. It's how they grow.

"Take these to the Rutkouskys, the Snyders and the Warzalas. Come right back when you're done. Got it?" Kerry said. It was an easy first assignment: Jillian wouldn't even have to cross the street.

"Got it," said Jillian. She stuffed the fliers in her pocket and made her way down the drive. Kerry made dinner.

Half an hour later, Kerry noticed Jillian wasn't home. Kerry reacted the way most mothers of first-graders would in that situation. She panicked. She called Denice Rutkousky. "Has Jillian been there?"

"Yes."

"Is she there now?"

"No. She left 20 minutes ago."

The Snyders. They lived one house down the street, to the left. "Did Jillian come by?"

"She did."

"Still there?"

"Not in the last 15 minutes."

Kerry's heart played bongos in her chest. "The first time I let her out of my sight . . ."

Her fingers shook as she dialed the home of the Warzalas, two houses up the street. If Jillian wasn't there, the next call would be to 9-1-1. The phone rang. Once, twice, three times. Oh, no.

That's when Jillian answered the Warzalas' phone.

"Jillian?"

"Yeah?"

"What are you doing?"

"Waiting for the Warzalas to get home."

Kerry wondered how Jillian got in. Wasn't their front door locked?

"Yeah," Jillian said. "I go 'round back."

Jillian had felt a sworn duty to place the invitation directly into the hands of Cathi Warzala. This was her first assignment out of the front yard. She wasn't going to blow it. She figured she'd just hang out in the Warzalas' family room until they showed up. She had her feet up in a La-Z-Boy. She was looking for some microwave popcorn. She really was.

"You can come home now," Kerry managed. All parents recognize that unusual mixture of anger and relief upon locating a wayward child. That was Kerry at that moment.

"Mrs. Warzala not home yet," Jillian protested.

"Home," said Kerry. "Now."

When Jillian arrived, Kerry didn't yell.

But I did. I yelled, and I lectured.

"Did Mom tell you to come right home?" I asked.

"I want to give Mrs. Warzala the note," said Jillian.

I went on a while, suggesting that the mailbox would have worked, that Mom was frantic.

"Fran-stick?" Jillian interjected.

. . . that if we were ever going to trust her to leave the yard, she had to do better, and that if she pulled that stunt again, I'd personally chain her to her bedpost for the rest of her life. The usual stuff.

I might have raised my voice above acceptable conversational levels.

Jillian listened calmly. She might even have nodded once or twice, in response to the obligatory "Do you understand me?" I could tell she was not moved by the force of my argument or by the logic involved. Jillian, who was by then 50 pounds of iron will, still believed she had been right to take up residence in the Warzala family room.

When I was done haranguing, or when she believed I was done, Jillian screwed up her face and looked at me dead-on.

"You wanna piece of me?" she asked.

"I beg your pardon?"

"You wanna piece of me, Daddy-O?"

I have no idea where she came up with that. Maybe it was from the movie *Home Alone,* which she and Kelly had seen, oh, 500 times. Maybe it was from one of Kelly's old videotapes of the *Teenage Mutant Ninja Turtles.* Maybe she'd heard it from some kid at school.

Regardless, I couldn't stay mad, even as I wanted to. "You better hope I don't want a piece of you," I managed.

"Come on," Jillian suggested.

I burst out laughing. Any groundwork I'd laid about coming home at the appointed time, and the penalties for failing to do so, was in a shambles.

I love Jillian's sense of humor, and I know you can't be funny without being smart. She may not be smart in the IQ sense. No one's suggesting Jillian will be building reactors anytime soon. But she's plenty smart in knowing what resonates. She understands what prompts a chuckle, what makes the synapses gather and fire.

This is essential to getting along with the world. Jillian is a citizen in good standing, not because she practices the King's English. Sometimes, even Kerry and I have to ask her to repeat herself. She gets along because she knows how to get along. She is social because she is confident in herself. She is confident because she has been placed in typical social situations and has succeeded.

Her sense of humor has eased her road. It is one of life's ordinary blessings.

This Deliver-the-Fliers Incident helped Jillian over whatever qualms she had about venturing beyond the demilitarized zone of the front yard. And the more we let her, the more that independence dynamic kept kicking in. All manner of interesting things ensued.

THERE ARE FOUR HOUSES on our little drive. At one time or another, small children were living in each one. Part of the drive's appeal was that parents could let their little ones out without worrying about traffic. So we let Jillian out. It was like letting a monkey loose into the people portion of the zoo.

One summer day, as the mothers of the drive gathered on folding chairs and the kids played, Jillian ventured unnoticed down to the Slatterys'. They had two kids—Kate the eldest and Tommy the youngest. Not that it mattered; Jillian was friends with everyone—whether they were interested or not.

Their storm door was open, so she walked inside. Maybe she called for Kate or Tommy. Maybe she just wanted to come in. When she discovered nothing or no one on the first floor that interested her, she went upstairs, and into the master bedroom, where she saw John Slattery emerge from the shower, seeking a towel.

"Hi, Mr. Slattery," Jillian said.

"Uh . . ." was the essence of John's comeback.

It might have been that same summer that Jillian stole a car.

The phone rang in the middle of the day. Kerry answered.

The man on the phone lived up the street, maybe five houses away. He didn't sound angry, really. Nor especially concerned. You could tell by his voice that he was talking while smiling. He knew Jillian. Or at least knew of her. She was the kid who had walked in on the naked guy.

"Your daughter took my son's Jeep out of our driveway," he said. "She's on Ashire, heading up to the pool."

The Jeep in question was electric and no bigger than a little red wagon. Ashire Lane was on the way to the neighborhood pool. I guess Jillian didn't feel like hitchhiking. By the time Kerry discovered our young car thief, Jillian was almost to the pool, steady-truckin' at about a mile an hour. "Does this Jeep belong to you?" Kerry asked.

"Yes," Jillian said.

"Jillian."

"I bought it."

She meant to say she "borrowed" the ride. At least that was my interpretation. Bought, borrowed. Whatever.

"I ride," Jillian added. She was pleased with herself.

Lots of Jillian's adventures provoked terror before laughter. She had a tendency to wander. Every other kid explored. In Jillian's mind, she was just doing what her peers did. In fifth grade, she decided it would be a great idea if she walked home from school. It might have been, but we lived eight miles from school.

By this time, Kerry had started back coaching high school girls' soccer in the fall. After Jillian's school day ended, she could take the regular school bus home. Or she could catch the bus that went from her school to the high school. That bus served kids involved in extracurriculars at the high school. Jillian was marginally a ball girl for the soccer team, though it was up to her if she came to practice or went straight home.

The bus drivers looked after her. They had walkie-talkies

and one of their daily routines at 2:30 p.m. was to check with each other, to make sure Jillian was on someone's bus. This particular day, she wasn't. The drivers called the school, then Kerry. The school dispatched its police officer to locate Jillian. Officer Fred Barnes set out in his cruiser, and it didn't take him long to find our world-trekking daughter. She was less than a mile from school. Amazingly, she was headed in the right direction.

"Jillian," said Officer Barnes. "I need to get you back to school, honey."

"No," Jillian said.

"C'mon, Jillian. Your mom's worried about you."

"I can't get in the car with you. My mom told me never ride with strangers."

Officer Barnes wasn't a stranger. Jillian knew him well. Jillian knew everybody well.

Fred finally convinced Jillian to climb aboard.

Jillian didn't limit her explorations to the home zip code. We spent a vacation one summer in a cottage on a pond, on Cape Cod. The house was secluded, right on the water. Maybe a half mile away, up a dirt road lined with pine trees, was the main road, a busy two-lane. There was a convenience store across the two-lane.

One fine very early morning, as Kerry, Kelly and I slept, Jillian arose with the idea that we needed doughnuts, and we needed them now. She knew just where to find them because she and Kelly had walked to the store the day before. She left with a dime and a nickel in her pocket. Nobody heard her.

We flew into mass panic when we woke up. Jillian was at the store when we found her, trying to negotiate down the price of a dozen doughnuts. Apparently, we'd gone from overly protective parents to parents whose daughter should have become a ward of the state. She'd have been in better hands.

These were times when Jillian's disability earned her a pass. Another child found tooling up the road in someone else's toy Jeep might have faced more severe consequences. A typical eight-year-old finding herself uninvited in a strange house, face-to-torso with a naked guy, might have lost dessert privileges or something. Probably, in our ever-quest for Jillian to be seen as typical, we should have punished her accordingly.

During the scary times, we let our hearts skip a beat, then we laughed. We laughed in the way other parents would laugh in the retelling of an incident that might have occurred several years earlier. We didn't tolerate Jillian's occasional excursions off the ranch. We didn't condone thievery or breaking and entering. She just didn't suffer the consequences Kelly would have.

Kids are kids. Innocence doesn't discriminate.

Jillian learned in school that you dial 9-1-1 if there's an emergency. In one particular instance, her emergency was that she needed some chocolate milk. I was out of town, thank God. Kerry was extremely surprised to see two police cars, lights flashing, in the driveway.

"Jillia-n-n-n!"

Afterward, we couldn't figure what she'd been most sorry about: That she'd called 9-1-1 for a frivolous reason. Or that the officers didn't have her chocolate milk.

Jillian also had a lemonade stand. On a day when no one was buying, she drew letters on cut-up pieces of notebook paper and put them in an envelope. Then she went to the

Whites' house (down the drive, on the right) and offered them the whole alphabet, at ten cents a letter.

Other life events prompted a more serious approach. Jillian hit puberty at age 11, in fourth grade. She had her first period on Christmas Day. This was one area in which Jillian was not delayed. When she noticed the discharge, she screamed for Kerry to come upstairs. "I think I having a baby," Jillian said.

Kerry told her what was happening and what it meant, the first of many talks regarding womanhood and the responsibility it entailed. I was delightedly out of that loop. I'd bought Kelly a jock strap, way back, when such accoutrements still existed. That was the extent of my involvement in matters that make men itch.

"You're a woman now," Kerry told Jillian.

A few days later, they went to a restaurant for lunch. Being small in stature, Jillian was often given a children's menu without being asked. But this day, the server did ask.

"And would you be needing a children's menu?"

"No," Jillian said. "I'm a woman now."

After Christmas break, Jillian returned to school with what she called her "woman thing"—a sanitary pad—packed in a lunch bag. One day, she asked to go to the restroom, knowing she needed to change her pad. "I have a 'mergency," she'd announced.

Problem was, she'd left it in the classroom. After several minutes, she hadn't returned. An anxious Nancy Croskey went to the bathroom, seeking Jillian.

"You okay, Jillian?" she asked.

"Yeah," Jillian answered. "But I need my pad."

She was developing her own personality. It was a unique

set of traits that reinforced the fact that Jillian was far more like us than not. Like her mom, Jillian loved to go out to eat. If restaurants were the New World, Kerry would be Columbus. We were running errands one Saturday at close to lunchtime when the subject of food came up.

"McDonald's," Jillian said.

"We're not going out to eat," I said.

"Applebee's," Jillian said. I told her we had food at home.

"Chili's," Jillian said. This was a child who was "cognitively delayed"?

"Burger King. Arby's, Frisch's, Wendy's." She proceeded to name every restaurant that had a kitchen. Free verse, with a drive-thru. "Outback, Johnny Rocket's, Steak-n-Shake, Penn Station, Domino's, Papa John's!"

She was very proud of herself.

Sometimes, we didn't know quite what to make of Jillian's progress. In ninth grade, a classmate had been giving her a hard time. Jillian almost never encountered meanness at school. Her classmates were universally kind, if mostly distant. But this time, one boy was not.

After a while, Jillian decided she'd heard enough. She passed the boy a note that the teacher intercepted.

"You're a deck," she'd written.

Now, typically, a parent wouldn't greet that with a smile, let alone the big laugh I let out when I heard what had happened. We're pretty sure Jillian wasn't calling the kid "a floor-like surface wholly or partially occupying one level of a hull, superstructure, or deckhouse." She was referring to a portion of his anatomy.

We were upset about that, sort of. We know high school

kids can't go around calling each other decks. But we were darned proud that Jillian was able to offer it in a complete and cogent (if misspelled) thought. And the thought she'd had was entirely "typical" for a ninth-grader.

Around that time, Jillian visited Kerry's sister in Baltimore. Janis had been recently divorced, which saddened Jillian. "I love my uncle Marc," she said, when she was told about the breakup. Jillian's way of consoling Janis was to offer to help make dinner. "My world-famous pasta salad" was to be Jillian's contribution.

Jan had company for dinner that night. "You can make this if you have a husband, or if you don't," Jillian announced.

The house Jan lived in was for sale at the time, and as Janis showed the place to a prospective buyer, Jillian said, "She used to have a husband, but not anymore." To which the bemused visitor responded, "Been there, honey."

Jillian's ability to provoke laughter was entirely without guile. The innocence of the acts gave the comedy a spontaneous purity that underscored its authenticity. It wasn't a performance. Jillian didn't try to make us laugh. She was just Jillian. Her eagerness to stretch came with its own challenges. It would also expand her choices, in all the ways Kerry and I had hoped.

Meantime, we send our sincerest apologies to The Deck, and to the owner of the Jeep. And to John Slattery. Jillian didn't mean anything by it. Really.

CHAPTER 9

Nancy

Education is not preparation for life.
Education is life itself.
—JOHN DEWEY

Jillian's earliest sessions with Martha showed us how eager she was to learn. Jillian wanted to keep up. Once she enrolled in school, the trick was finding teachers who would mine that eagerness.

When Jillian was two years old, Kerry enrolled her in sort of a pre-preschool that was for kids with special needs. It offered the rudimentaries—sitting up straight, holding silverware, mixing with peers—but more than anything the school showed us what we did not want for Jillian: A school strictly for special-needs children. After that, Jillian spent the next three years in typical preschool, and she loved it. She'd be the first one up in the morning, getting herself ready to go. Pencils packed, scissors stowed, teachers' names memorized.

"Today, I see Miss Jackie," she'd say. Her brother thought she was strange.

Jillian was able to keep up for those three years. She adapted easily. In the world of crayons and paste, aptitude wasn't a concern. Jillian knew what everyone else knew: Letters. Numbers. Colors. How to get along. She got along well. She loved being there. We were convinced that Jillian and teachers would be the perfect match of energy and idealism. Armed with this pleasant naïveté, we enrolled her in kindergarten when she was almost six years old.

The year before, Kerry had met with the school psychologist at Loveland Elementary, the local public grade school. She wanted to make sure the proper authorities knew Jillian was arriving next September and that a support staff understood that they would need to set aside extra time to provide Jillian with the extra help she would require. At least that was the plan. Immediately we faced resistance.

Loveland Elementary had what it called a "unit classroom" set up specifically for special-needs students. It was in the windowless basement of the school, segregated metaphorically and otherwise. "The regular-ed teacher might not want Jillian," an administrator said.

"You tell the regular-ed teacher it's the law," Kerry shot back. She'd attended workshops on this very topic for a few years. Kerry knew what she knew.

This was the first time we demanded that Jillian be fully included in regular education classrooms. That's school-speak for, "We want our daughter to be given the same schooling, in the same setting, as every other kid. If you resist, we'll whack you with the rule book."

We wanted Jillian to grow as much socially as academically. Our belief was that she needed to have typical peers as her guides, and through them she would learn the classroom do's and don't's. We also wanted her to get as much book learning as she could. We didn't see the point of putting her in a segregated class, where much of the modeling she'd be receiving was of behaviors we didn't want. Children with Down syndrome don't develop socially as quickly as typical kids. Jillian was already doing well socially. We didn't want to slow that development by having her in a segregated classroom.

Kids watch each other. How they behave, what they wear, what movies and music they like. Peer influence is more powerful than anything a parent can offer. If you want kids with disabilities to achieve beyond the norm, why would you put them in a segregated classroom, only with other kids with disabilities? We didn't know why anyone would want that. This was 1995, not 1955.

In 1975, Congress passed the Individuals with Disabilities Education Act (IDEA). It was a monumental civil rights triumph for kids who wanted to be in typical classrooms, learning and socializing with their typical peers. What *Brown v. Board of Education* had done for African Americans, IDEA established for children with disabilities. IDEA made it law that children with disabilities must receive a "free and appropriate" education in the "least restrictive environment," and that guides—known as Individualized Education Plans—be developed to meet their specific needs. Jillian began her first year of kindergarten with an IEP.

And that was the beginning of our grand experiment.

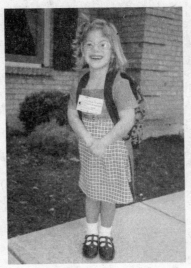

The first day of first grade.

Charlene Green was Jillian's kindergarten teacher entirely by chance. The second of Jillian's guardian angels had appeared. We knew of her reputation as a stern, respected educator whose emphasis on reading fit perfectly with what we wanted for our daughter. Charlene didn't know Jillian. In fact, she'd taught for 29 years in the Loveland school system and had never had a child with Down syndrome.

Charlene wanted Jillian in her classroom, though. She was intrigued and concerned. She had no idea how it might turn out. Neither did we. Preschool had been half a day, and though learning was involved, it wasn't stressed. The social aspect was more important. Kindergarten would be different. Kids would begin in earnest the lifelong learning process. Reading, writing, adding and subtracting. How would Jillian do?

Kerry met with Charlene shortly before school started and came away elated. This, she said, was a teacher whose philosophy was aligned with ours. Jillian's exuberance and fearlessness were going to find the ideal task master. Charlene would teach the lion. And tame her a little.

"You're in my room, you will be reading before you leave," Charlene told Kerry. "Jillian will be a student, same as any other child in my classroom. I'm going to teach her the same way I teach everyone else. I will expect her to achieve to her potential."

Amen. Jillian had a teacher who would respect what she was capable of doing. That's all we'd ever ask. It's all we ever wanted. Allowances would be made. Jillian would have an aide. But expectations would abide. In Charlene Green's kindergarten class, Jillian would learn the proper way to hold a pencil and a pair of scissors. She would improve upon what she'd gathered in preschool. Most essentially, she would begin to learn to read.

Charlene produced for Jillian the building blocks of reading: "There is just one way to teach children to read," she explained. "You know your letters, you know your sounds. You know your phonetic rules. And you repeat them, until you get it right."

This was all vital. But equally important was the attitude with which Charlene made it happen. No patronizing, no short cuts. Expect, don't accept.

After a year in Charlene's class, Jillian was close to reading—close enough that Charlene recommended Jillian spend another year in her room. The school administrators were not receptive to this. They didn't say it. But it was clear to us they thought "flunking" Jillian would look bad on their record.

What they said was they were worried that going forward Jillian would be too old for her grade level. She'd be an eight-year-old in first grade. Too advanced physically, they said. This was so obviously contrived that when we met to discuss it, I couldn't help myself and said: "So your biggest fear in Jillian's education is that she will have breasts before anyone else."

Jillian got a second year in Charlene's class, and she entered first grade knowing how to read.

Those first few years of school were not a struggle—for us or for Jillian. We nagged on the edge of being overly insistent with everyone who had a hand in Jillian's education. There were school people who didn't welcome our presence; at least that was how we felt. No one was overtly resistant, or even unkind. They were just glad when Jillian advanced from their building and into the next one. Generally, we got along, mostly through the benevolence of the teachers themselves.

In elementary school, the kids don't switch classes. The teachers have the same group of 25 or 30 for the whole year. They get to know their students. This was especially important with Jillian. Her teachers could view her as a special kid, not just a kid with special needs. Perception is reality. Jillian was always good at making positive perceptions.

IN MARCH 1990, FIVE months after Jillian's birth, I wrote a cover story about her for *Cincinnati* magazine. I'd met the editor at a civic function. She'd heard about Jillian. Everybody had heard about Jillian. Cincinnati is a small place. After the usual awkward expressions of condolence, congratulation and encouragement, the editor asked if I'd explain to her readers what it "really" felt like to be the father a child with Down syndrome.

I wrote about athletes for a living. Their efforts are uncomplicated and easily described. They win, they lose, they make lots of money. This was different. It was raw and personal. I didn't hesitate to accept the assignment. I did wonder what I'd say, and how I'd say it. My first thought when asked what it "really" felt like was *Compared to what?* So I just said it. I wrote 3,000 words in half a day. They roared like the last wild river. The story I offered was a full-blown catharsis. It was tears on a page:

> We had been denied the most passionate event of life, the birth of a healthy child. Jillian is a joy, a treasure, a miracle. And she breaks our hearts every day.

Right after Jillian's birth, what I saw as a wound was too raw for me to assess reasonably. The self-woe flowed:

> Jillian is only (five) months old. I can't help feeling her best steps were stolen away from her, before she ever got to the dance . . .
> I wonder if, some enchanted evening, my daughter will know the smell of a boyfriend's cologne . . .
> Is the fog lifting, or simply gathering silently for a lifetime encore?

The article ended on a hopeful note—*"We want her to be productive, respected and fulfilled. We don't care if she can be a singer. We just want her to be able to sing"*—even though its overall tone reflected an abiding sadness.

One of the people who read *Cincinnati* magazine and saw the cover with Kerry, me, and a big-eyed baby in a pink sleeper, staring right at the camera, was Nancy Croskey. It was a happy coincidence that Nancy taught fourth grade in our school district. The day she read the magazine story she became determined to have Jillian in her class. She saw something in that little girl. Maybe it was a memory of how hard her own early school experience had been. Maybe she remembered a caring teacher from her own childhood who had helped her get through some bad times. Perhaps Nancy Croskey talked to Charlene Green. Regardless, Nancy embraced Jillian as no one had before.

Nancy had been teaching for more than two decades when a tiny, enthusiastic child walked into her classroom, lugging a backpack that hung from her shoulders to the backs of her knees.

"I'm Jillian," Jillian announced.

"I know," Nancy said.

What Nancy didn't know then was that everything she'd experienced in her life before that moment had prepared her for what was about to happen in Room 36 at Loveland Elementary School. Nancy wanted to be a teacher who makes a difference? Well, here was your difference—all three feet eight inches of her, standing in your doorway, carrying a house on her back.

What happened in the next ten months was a collaboration of hearts and minds. Two people shared what was best about each other. When it was finished, both would be changed profoundly. Congress created IDEA so that relationships could form, like the one between Jillian and Mrs. Croskey. Opportunity met burden, and found it light.

WHEN NANCY CROSKEY WAS in the sixth grade, her teacher said to her, in front of her classmates, "You're not as smart as your brother."

But Nancy was smart, even if her intelligence was tucked away, inside her shyness, buried beneath an inability to comprehend what she read. She dreaded being embarrassed in front of the class. "I was a slow learner," she recalls. "If I were in school now, I'd be on an IEP."

She knew all the words, and she could pronounce them. She could watch them and study them and roll them across her tongue until they emerged as speech, whole and perfect sounding. It was a grand illusion; Nancy didn't know what the words meant. Children laughed at her, and that was terrifying.

This wasn't limited to reading books. Nancy got lost on math problems that involved words. "If Johnny went to school with three cookies in his lunch bag, and gave away two . . ." Dread arrived in first or second grade when Nancy was made to read aloud to her classmates, and was then asked to describe what she'd just read. "I was humiliated," Nancy recalls.

This smart, underachieving little girl began to fear school, until she found an ally in third grade. A teacher she remembers only as Mrs. Daniels recognized her limitations. What previous teachers had seen as a burden, Mrs. Daniels regarded as a chance. She didn't make Nancy read aloud. She could tell that Nancy was a visual learner.

Mrs. Daniels taught her multiplication with numbered magnets affixed to a wall. Nancy could understand what she saw. Mrs. Daniels chose books that partnered pictures with the words to further the story. If Nancy could see an idea, she could remember it and express it.

Mrs. Daniels didn't have all the answers, though. Nancy continued to struggle. Homework meant hours at night at the kitchen table, grinding, hoping for magic that would make the words have meaning. Her father was patient and insistent, hammering home the essentials of geometry and Stephen Crane. It was sometimes 11:00 p.m. by the time Nancy had finished her homework. Or it had finished her. None of this fazed her father. "Okay," he'd say. "Get the book and do it again."

Starting in third grade, Nancy realized she could learn. The way she learned was different. "It isn't one size fits all. Children are individuals," Nancy says.

Caring teachers could teach her. Nancy didn't become a teacher because she intended to change lives. She remembered how hard school had been for her, and she simply wanted to make it easier for those she taught. Her aspirations found a perfect partner in Jillian, whose natural perk and sass worked well in a place where kids were still too young to judge someone harshly just because they didn't quite look like they did. At Loveland Intermediate School, Jillian became known as The Mayor.

I saw it up close. My odd sportswriter hours allowed me time to help in her classroom. When the class took breaks, to go to the library or for lunch or recess, I'd walk with Jillian through the halls. Every kid, every teacher and all of the administrators said hello to her. And she knew all of their names.

"Hi, Allison."

"Hi, Jillian."

"Hi, Brandon."

"Hi, Jillian."

"How do you know everyone's name?" I asked her.

"They're my friends," Jillian said.

The principal, Mr. Brooks, and her second-grade teacher,

Mrs. Burke. Andy B and Andy J. Sarah and Sara, the secretaries in the office. The custodian. No one escaped Jillian's recognition and acknowledgment. Occasionally, she would request a bathroom break. If she didn't return right away, her teacher sent another student to look for her. Jillian would be in the gym, talking to Mr. McCoy, the phys ed teacher.

Nancy Croskey may have been shy when she was young, but this kid who needed five minutes to ditch the womb never had that problem. Between classes, she'd walk the halls, singing that Britney Spears song about Oops and doing it again. She'd invite all of her friends to dance with her.

Jillian's issues were of intellect, not reticence. Her eagerness to learn was innate. It worked in tune with her desire to please. Jillian never wanted to let anyone down. From Mrs. Croskey, she got the help and extra support she needed. And in turn Mrs. Croskey observed in Jillian a spirit she'd always hoped to see in her students. She admired Jillian's tenacity, and her ability to relate to other kids. Jillian celebrated her own successes, but no more than everyone else's. She congratulated her classmates when they did well. She reassured them when they didn't.

Jillian never had a bad day. She might start out a little down, but it never lasted. Nancy said Jillian "had that spunkiness about her. She never said I can't do that. She would try anything. She wanted to be a part of everything."

Not everything was easy. Homework was a nightly bang at a wall. The simplest of problems—two-plus-two, literally and figuratively—could be a mystery to Jillian. Sometimes all she had was her will, and sometimes that wasn't enough.

Jillian was usually the first to arrive in Room 36, straight from the school bus. She would heave her backpack—WHAM!!—onto a table "Homework not so good," Jillian would say. "I bring a note from Dad."

Dad might have spent an hour the night before, searching for word definitions or the proper formula to solve a math problem. He might have had trouble with the instructions, or he might have found the clues in Jillian's assignment book less than helpful. Dad might have been frustrated or annoyed or, more likely, a combination. Dad might have slung a few choice words not heard in church. Lots of nights Dad and Jillian were two people in darkness, searching for the damned flashlight.

"My dad was mad," Jillian would say. "I don't want my dad to be mad at me. I try my hardest."

"Don't worry about it," Nancy would say. "We'll find a better way to do it. And your dad's not mad at you."

Sufficiently soothed, Jillian would rummage through her backpack, locate her lunch bag, and comment on what Kerry or I had packed for her. "Carrot sticks again," she'd say.

With help from classroom aide Mary Smethurst, Nancy taught Jillian. Spelling words, simple math, who lives in the White House. Nancy's own experience told her that Jillian was a visual learner and suggested we use index cards for Jillian's vocabulary words. On one card, the word; on another, its definition. Six or eight words a week, cards and definitions arrayed across the kitchen table. Jillian matched the words with their definitions.

A few years earlier, we'd started playing a child's version of Concentration. Kerry or I would pick eight pairs from a deck of cards, shuffle them, then place them facedown on the table, in four rows of four. We'd take turns with Jillian, trying to match the pairs. More often than not, Jillian would win. She learned visually, the same as her teacher had, three decades earlier.

We also started to realize how Jillian's presence had a positive impact on the other kids. They liked her. She was kind.

One day, Nancy decided the class would bake a cake together. It combined cooking skills with math know-how as well as the importance of reading and understanding the directions. One of Jillian's friends, a boy named Layton, had never cooked. He had been homeschooled, Nancy said. "He'd never so much as cracked an egg." Well, that day Layton broke a few eggs. On the floor. He became frustrated, angry and was crying.

"I show you," Jillian said to him.

"What?"

"I show you."

Jillian cracked the egg on the side of the bowl. It slid into the cake mix. "Like that," she said. "You try, Layton."

Nancy never eased up. She could be as stubborn as Jillian was. "I treated her the way I treated all the kids," Nancy said. "I would introduce a unit and point out the key things I wanted her to get out of it. I wanted her to know the three branches of government. I'd write them on the blackboard, I'd show her pictures."

The White House, the Capitol building, the Supreme Court.

Nancy modified the work for Jillian. She increased the type size and included more picture clues. Jillian rewarded those efforts with a determination to get everything right. Nothing was too hard for her. Jillian would try everything. She would never say she couldn't do something.

All year, Nancy pushed gently, and Jillian responded. The collaboration produced wins on both sides. Nancy taught Jillian, and Jillian returned the favor. "How can that not affect you, when you have this fourth-grader who thinks nothing's impossible?" Nancy said. "There are teachers that celebrate having kids like Jillian. I think you have to have a kid like Jillian in your classroom, to open your eyes to what's possible."

I'd always believed teachers were noble people, and that teaching was a noble calling. Long hours, low pay, vital jobs. In a perfect world, teachers would be millionaires, and ballplayers would make $50,000 a year. Teachers would live in big houses and drive expensive cars. Ballplayers would buy their uniforms and pack their lunches in Tupperware. Our public education system rests on the hope that teachers enter the profession with an eye on making a difference. They mold minds and shape lives, one Dick and Jane reader at a time. To believe otherwise is to entrust our children to people who are in it for the summers off and the generous retirement plans.

There was not a better child than Jillian to determine which ones were which.

"When school again?" she'd ask, on a Friday.

"Monday," we'd answer.

"When dat?"

"After Saturday and Sunday."

"I love my school."

Jillian and Nancy have remained best friends, even as Jillian has gotten too old for Nancy's classroom. They go shopping. They go out to eat. They talk on the phone. They exchange gifts on their birthdays. Lately, Nancy has advocated for Jillian to get her driver's license, an almost unheard-of achievement for a person with Down syndrome. Not long ago, Nancy arrived at their dinner date with a copy of the Ohio driver's manual.

Nancy champions Jillian, and Jillian lifts up Nancy. They teach each other. "She brought everything to our relationship. I got more from it than she got from me. Jillian knows the important stuff," Nancy said.

The miracle of a teacher is that person's ability to bend a life toward good. The reward for that is to know a person like Jillian. An education for each. Life itself.

CHAPTER 10

The Battleground of Dreams

*The special education law doesn't say we're supposed
to provide an optimal education. It says we're
supposed to provide a free and
appropriate education.*
—KEVIN BOYS, FORMER LOVELAND SCHOOLS
SUPERINTENDENT

*The reasonable man adapts himself to the world.
The unreasonable one persists in trying to
adapt the world to himself.*
—GEORGE BERNARD SHAW

Kevin Boys says the term "Public Law 94-142" "just rolls off
the tongue." That's the formal name for IDEA, the Individuals
with Disabilities Education Act. Congress passed the law right
after Boys graduated from high school, and before he attended
college with a career in public education his goal. Before this

law was passed in 1975, one million kids with disabilities in the United States were denied any public education; four million more were segregated from their non-disabled peers, in a sort of out-of-sight, out-of-mind purgatory. In the land of the free, these kids wore chains. They had no chance.

Thanks to IDEA, every child would be invited to the learning dance. It was a good deal in 1975 because it pulled back the curtain on the shamefully narrow vision we'd had for our citizens with disabilities. Its principles gave birth to the "Expect, Don't Accept" way Kerry and I would approach Jillian's life. Jillian would not be Jillian without IDEA. Because of it, Jillian would have a chance.

Boys embraced the concept. "The vision in this country is that we educate all our kids," he said. It was also a topic of debate whenever Loveland schools needed to pass a levy. Some parents who didn't have kids with special needs questioned the district's expenditures in that area. Boys usually responded by saying, "This is the greatest country on earth, because we have decided all children deserve an education." It was more than just a good idea, Boys said. "It's one of those moral imperatives that sets us apart as a country."

But this moral imperative got lost sometimes and was detoured into a school conference room, where it was fought over by two groups of people who supposedly shared the goal of getting a child educated. The problem was that each side came with its own notions of how that would happen. Often what Kerry and I wanted for Jillian differed so much from what the school people desired that it seemed as if we were speaking English and they were hearing Chinese.

No parents of typical kids have to fight their school district for the right to have their children in a typical classroom. They don't concern themselves with the stereotypes and perceptions some of their children's teachers have of students with disabilities. But a quarter century after IDEA became law, we were still convincing school people of its worth. Imagine black Americans in 1989, 25 years after passage of the Civil Rights Act, fighting for a seat at the front of a public bus.

Any child with disabilities who enters the school systems is given an Individualized Education Plan (IEP), which is a road map that describes what that child's needs are. The IEP sets "reasonable" learning goals, and it states what the schools will do to attain them. Parents and school people design it together, agree on what is to be done, and how. In our case, the school people were to bring the dedication and skills while Kerry and I were to supply the support and the trust.

Kumbayas all around. That's the theory.

In practice, an IEP meeting can feel like a divorce settlement hearing, without the consensus of a divorce. The two sides sit apart from each other, on opposite sides of a long, rectangular conference table in a room with no windows. On their side is an army of counselors, teachers, therapists, a school psychologist and administrators of all stripes. On our side was basically Kerry and I.

Some of the people on the other side know Jillian. Most do not. Some see working with her as an opportunity to pursue a calling; some see Jillian as an itch they'd rather not scratch. But as long as Jillian was in this school, we were stuck with each other. I always wanted to pull out a photo of Jillian and put it on the table. I'd say, "This is who we're here for today. Do you know Jillian? Have you met her? She loves school. Did you know that? She works hard. She isn't a concept or a philosophy or a line item. She's a child. Please see her as such, and educate her the way the law says you have to."

It wasn't about money. Issues of funding didn't come up until high school, when Jillian needed services the school couldn't provide. It was about perceptions. Could Jillian learn? How much could she learn? Is the attempt worthwhile?

Once teachers and aides became comfortable with Jillian, those questions were easily answered. Getting them to that point was the challenge. Don't look at Jillian. See her.

When you're trying to get your child a "free and appropriate" education, perceptions are everything. They are the first line of resistance, the last line and everything in between. Educating the educators became central. This isn't 1965. It's not just a moral imperative. It's the law.

Teachers are no different than the rest of us who might have been doing something a certain way for a long while. They're resistant to change. They've taught a certain way, with a class full of typical kids, and they don't like being told how to do their jobs.

They resist because, as Nancy Croskey suggested, "Some of the younger teachers think of it as an easy way to earn a living. They don't want to ruffle feathers. They do what they're told." Nancy also believed that special-ed teachers "pigeonhole kids like Jillian. They set goals that were too low, because they knew they could reach them."

After Jillian finished fourth grade, she would go into a new building for fifth grade, and again the district wanted to place her in a special-ed unit classroom. Unit classrooms were a relic from the 1960s. The belief was they made it easier to "manage" "those" children if they were all in one group. Little consideration was given to the fact that they would receive a lesser chance to learn academically or they would miss out on being integrated into the school culture as a whole. Unit classrooms were easy and cost efficient. There was no need to "bother" classroom teachers with kids with special needs.

During the summer before fifth grade, Kerry and Nancy Croskey met with the intermediate school principal and the special-education teacher. Nancy argued that Jillian had to be in the regular classroom. "Not just for her sake," she said, "but for yours, too. You'd be doing a disservice to your teachers, and to the rest of your students, not to include Jillian in their classrooms. It will make them better teachers. It will make your students better people."

Nancy was persuasive. Jillian would be in the regular-ed classroom.

Meantime, the IEP meetings with Jillian's "team" of teachers and aides continued. We'd meet in the spring, to set the goals for the next year. We'd meet again in the fall, to make sure everything was in order. We'd meet other times, too, when Kerry and I had issues. We had lots of issues.

We'd ask that homework assignments be modified so the amount of work was at a more manageable level for Jillian. We also requested that the classroom aide or the special-ed teacher amend the questions or problems to Jillian's aptitudes. What we got, generally, was less homework with the same degree of difficulty. If the rest of the class had ten questions, Jillian got six or seven. That's not modifying.

We'd beg that aides help Jillian with her assignment book, the paperback-size ringed binder that kept her day straight.

We asked them to go over it with her before she left for the day to make sure it was complete and accurate. Often, it was anything but. Jillian managed it herself most days.

"Did the teacher help you with this?" we might ask after looking at the assignment book at home.

"No," Jillian would say. "I do it myself."

Later, in high school, the aides often took Jillian out of the regular classroom and brought her into what was known as the "resource room" to work on classroom assignments. The resource room was a place for her to feel excluded. It was a place for students with special needs to be segregated from their typical peers. It was easier for the aides to work with Jillian there, apparently, though no explanations were ever offered. But it wasn't the law. It wasn't part of Jillian's IEP. Kerry and I had to insist that Jillian not be pulled from regular-ed classes.

We also requested that we be given a week's notice before major tests. That rarely happened. We asked that teachers provide a modified study guide for those tests. Generally, Kerry and I did the modifying. We'd send notes in with Jillian, asking teachers to do better. Sometimes, after a long and fruitless homework session, frustration would do me in. I'd write machine-gun blasts in the margins of the assignment book.

"DON'T UNDERSTAND THIS. NOT MODIFIED."

On other occasions, my notes would be longer, tamer and filled with begging:

"We want to help Jillian. She's eager to do the work. We need you to make sure her assignments are accurate and modified. Help us help her. Thank you."

Or, on nights when I simply wasn't in the mood:

"ANOTHER WASTED EVENING. PLEASE DO YOUR JOB."

It wasn't the hours required. It wasn't Jillian's lack of trying. It was the grinding exasperation that, seemingly, the teachers and the aides didn't understand what we needed. Or worse, didn't care.

I felt as if I were pushing the same boulders around the same room every night. Home should be a haven, where you go to escape the workday crush. For a few hours lots of week-day evenings, it was anything but.

Happily, it never affected the way we dealt with each other. If anything, the homework frustrations tightened our collective fist. We couldn't fight for Jillian if we fought each other. And since Jillian's education wasn't Kelly's concern, we didn't let our anger impact anything we did with him.

We coped by plowing ahead. We fed off Jillian's successes. Singular pursuits have no room for sideshows.

After a while, though, Kerry did wise up to my exasperation. She'd filter my anger. Or toss it away. "You can't say that," she'd say.

"The hell I can't."

"That isn't helping."

"It helps me," I'd say. "Besides, what is helping? We have the same discussion, over and over."

There were other things. The intermediate school didn't give Jillian a lock for her locker because they didn't think she could manage a combination. She went a few months with an unsecured locker until Kerry visited her and noticed it. Kerry requested a lock. We worked with Jillian for a few hours until she learned how to use it. This seems a small thing, one play early in the first inning of a baseball game. But when you're dealing with perceptions that need to be changed, a child without a lock for her locker represents the bottom of the ninth.

The constant push-pull served no one's needs. Months of frustration would gather and spill over at the IEP meetings. The meetings became a contrary mash of tension and tediousness. After a few minutes of introductory, forced politeness, we'd address the IEP itself. It was 12 pages of vague and obvious goals—"Jillian needs to fully and successfully participate in the general education classroom"—and concrete services that were often ignored: "Chapter outlines for Science, Social Studies and English provided at beginning of each unit (by regular teachers)." That kind of thing happened rarely, and usually only when we insisted.

Still, Kerry and I continued to attend the school meetings, and she had faith that the teachers would teach Jillian to the best of their abilities no matter what was written in the IEPs. They would challenge Jillian and set goals. We assumed that if she could handle more than the goal, they'd give her more.

Kerry didn't take the time to read and study the IEPs. She trusted. I didn't study them either. I trusted too. These IEPs were coma inducing. We trusted the school to do what it said it would do. It would follow the road map. It would alter the route when necessary. We assumed this. Jillian's elementary school experience suggested we should. That was a mistake.

As Jillian advanced to high school and tested far below grade level, Kerry went back through Jillian's IEPs for grades five through eight. What she discovered was that entire IEPs had stayed exactly the same from one year to the next. Not only weren't the teachers modifying tests and homework, they weren't revising the IEPs either. Nor did they ever take into account Jillian's achievement and deviate from what was in the IEP. The road map never changed even as new highways were built.

Jillian's teachers did what was easiest, not what was right. Least resistance was the preferred path. They took advantage of our trust. They stunted Jillian's education. They did it for years. It felt like a punch in the gut.

"I should have been more vigilant," Kerry said. Maybe so. But it wasn't our vigilance that needed to be questioned—it was our trust. We believed in teachers, partly because Kerry was one. She knew the challenges. "I realize there are only so many hours in a day," she said.

That wasn't it either. Time didn't shortchange Jillian. Attitudes did. The only time the shackles of perception—Can this child really learn at her grade level?—loosened was when Kerry and I were a perpetual pain in the ass at Loveland Intermediate. But it was a constant struggle, and the shackles never came off completely.

When Kevin Boys said, "By and large, school people are good people who want to do the right thing," we agreed. Why wouldn't they want to do right? As Boys added, "The person you're arguing with across the table has children, too."

Yes. But his child isn't my child. If that were so, chances are he'd be arguing and fighting on behalf of his child the same way I was. There was never anyone on our IEP team who had a child with an intellectual disability. No one walked with us on that path. I wonder how that might have changed things, if anything might have been different.

I was not George Bernard Shaw's "reasonable man." I fully

expected the world to adapt to me. I had the law on my side. Some parents of kids with special needs are grateful that their children are even in regular classrooms. I wasn't one of those parents. Neither was Kerry. We knew Jillian deserved better than she was getting. And we were right.

"Why don't you people simply obey the law?" I said during one IEP gathering.

"I don't think there's any call for argument," came the answer. "We all want what's best for Jillian."

"Then do it," I said.

That's when everyone would flip the page of the IEP, metaphorically flipping me off and returning to the tense and false civility that marked most of these meetings. It was always easier for the school people to hide behind vaguely de-fined "goals" than to actually defend their position, that Jillian couldn't learn to the extent we believed she could, so why try? Which, strictly speaking, was indefensible.

There was an ideal in all of this. As the IDEA ideal was originally conceived, it was supposed to look like this: Teach-ers and typical kids engage a child whose ability to learn was compromised in the womb. They come to realize that she takes longer to learn, to speak, to grasp. Being with Jillian is life in slow motion.

In return, they get a friend. Someone guaranteed never to judge them or make them feel small. Jillian's intellectual blinders allow only good thoughts. Her capacity for uplift was limited only by those who declined to embrace it. Jillian lived up to her end of the deal. She gave, freely. Teachers and peers never got cheated. They would come to understand that dif-ferent isn't bad.

Ideally, it's a good contract. Everybody wins. That was the argument Kerry and I would make, time after time at the meetings.

That's when someone would say, "Let's turn to page eight."

In Jillian's 16 years of education—counting preschool and two years of kindergarten—I never owned a firm grip on how lots of Jillian's teachers regarded her. Burden or opportunity? A willing participant in the learning experience? Or a drag on the day-to-day progress of the entire class of kids? It's unfair to say they all felt more burdened than enriched by having her in class. It's easy to say they didn't work hard enough. I'm not a teacher. I don't know the challenges they face every day.

I know my daughter though. I know the opportunities missed by teachers who thought she was burdensome. When her time was done, I credited her cap-and-gown moment as much to her as to the people to whom we'd lent her seven hours a day, five days a week.

When Congress passed IDEA in 1975, its members didn't envision this sort of showdown. They just wanted to give kids with disabilities a fighting chance. We fought, all right. After a few years of this, and certainly by the time Jillian was in high school, it became less about getting her the services to which she was entitled, and more about principle. It became about winning.

Education speaks to the heart of everything we wanted for Jillian. The fight to get her educated brought every element of dealing with a disabled individual into play. What we want for Jillian and what the world believes is possible are getting closer, but they're still not the same. Until we span that canyon, lots of people's talents will never be utilized fully.

This issue isn't only about kids with disabilities. It's about how perceptions limit or expand potential. Ask African Americans: How many of our citizens have been denied a chance to shine? How much light did the rest of us miss because of it?

Jillian was in the eye of it all, the most eager of students. On the morning of her last day of her fifth-grade year, Jillian sat at the kitchen table, pounding a bowl of Frosted Flakes. She was unusually quiet. I don't like morning. It's best not to speak to me before noon. Jillian never followed that rule. Most mornings, she was a rooster.

"What's up, Jills?" I asked.

"I know I'm weird," she said. "But I'm really gonna miss school."

CHAPTER 11

Homework

I am defeated all the time. Yet to victory I am born.
—RALPH WALDO EMERSON

Even during the worst of the IEP collisions, no one doubted Jillian's determination and effort. She'd inherited Kerry's steel will, and she had her own desire to make people happy. Nowhere was Jillian's school spirit more defined than at the homework table.

Homework became a metaphor for everything we were up against. We had demanded that she be fully included in regular-ed classrooms. Homework was the symbol, sometimes mocking us, that Jillian be given her rightful chance. So here she was, in the midst of a nightly homework morass. You asked for it . . .

Kerry and I felt a certain pressure to justify what we'd insisted on for Jillian, and at times we'd despair when it didn't work. Homework was the first line of resistance in a school system we were forcing to change. It was front and center in our ongoing battle to get Jillian the education to which she was entitled. Kerry and I were Daniel Boone. We were blazing trails at school. Homework was the bear in the woods.

Jillian's backpack was an impressive place. It was an exaggerated purse. Fossilized items—peanut butter and jelly sandwiches, for instance—could be found at the bottom. Anything a kid who loved school could ever possibly need was jammed into that stretched assemblage of nylon.

You could also count on finding various lunch accoutrements. I packed her lunch half the time, but that didn't stop Jillian from adding to the scripted menu. Oreos were a favorite as she got older, but there were potato chips and crackers of all sorts. At Halloween, all manner of bite-size teeth killers got in the bag. "I love my lunch," she explained. Jillian packed for school as if she were going on an eating vacation. And don't forget the miniature football, for recess with the guys. And a frame, containing a three-by-five-inch picture of Walker, our black Labrador retriever. "Why do you take a picture of Walker to school?" I asked.

"Because I love my Walker," Jillian said.

The backpack was so big, we worried about back pain. If Jillian weighed 85 pounds in fourth grade, 25 of them were owed to this appendage she yanked onto her shoulders. She looked like a mover hauling a refrigerator.

"Is that thing too heavy? Let's see what we can take out of there," I asked occasionally.

"It's fine, Dad. My 'portant stuff."

We pondered getting Jillian a small, wheeled suitcase, but we didn't know how she'd manage climbing the school bus steps. So we sent her off every morning with a refrigerator on her back. Pencils, pens, markers. Reams of notebook paper. A ruler, a big eraser. Why do you need a thousand sheets of paper? "For big mistakes," Jillian offered. Separate three-ring plastic folders for each subject. A hairbrush.

And an assignment book. That weighed the most. On all of us.

Every student had an assignment book for homework details. It was the size of a five-by-eight-inch book. Each lined page had a day and a date. All students were expected to write down their homework assignments; so was Jillian, though she often had help from an aide. Sometimes, the assignment book was perfect, the key to the homework highway for that particular night. On those days, each subject would be followed by a colon, then the pages to be read or the problems to be worked. Jillian had written it all in, in her diligent scrawl that was just legible enough. Just as often, the aide had done the writing. On those blessed nights, we could begin the homework task assured that we were doing the right work.

On other nights, the assignments would be wrong. On those nights, the assignment book assumed a life all its own. It was an evil existence, full of fear and dread and my four-letter frustrations that sometimes made Jillian cry. "The damned homework is hard enough when the assignment is right!" I'd say. "What is so (expletive) hard about an aide or a teacher looking at the (expletive) assignment, to make sure Jillian copied the (expletive) thing the right (expletive) way?"

All kids need help with homework sometimes. With Jillian, help with homework was an occupation that became a preoccupation that became an obsession that, on occasion, became a full-blown source of rage and doubting.

Kerry and I alternated homework nights, because after working all day ourselves, neither of us relished consecutive nights at the kitchen table. Kerry was far more patient than I, partly because she was a teacher and patience is a teacher's best friend. She was also more closely involved with Jillian's day-to-day learning and thus better equipped to deal with the setbacks.

I just got mad a lot.

"Whaddaya got?" I'd say.

Jillian would haul in the backpack, toss it onto the kitchen table, an act of physical strength and an unburdening.

"Math and vocab," she'd say.

"Lemme see the assignment book."

Jillian would scrape through the backpack and tentatively hand it over.

On the good nights, we'd start right away. "It says, 'Review vocab words for test Friday.' You got the words?"

There'd be more pawing, deep into the maw of the backpack, where she'd find 16 three-by-five index cards. Eight with words on them—eight with definitions. So far, so smooth.

Mary Smethurst had picked the words. Mary was Jillian's aide for three years, grades two through four. Caring, empathetic and kind, Mary became the engine of Jillian's aspirations. If Jillian was able to learn something, Mary would see that she did. She wrote the vocabulary words on one side of the index card. Sometimes, on the other side, she'd draw a picture to illustrate the word. We'd look up the word, then write its definition on a separate card.

This side of the kitchen table: Words.

That side: Definitions. It was like when we played Concentration with playing cards.

"You ready?" I'd say.

Jillian was always ready. She was born ready. "Of course," she'd answer.

"Challenge," I said. A fitting word to start with, I thought.

"Change," Jillian said.

"No, sweetie. ChaLLenge." I'd press the tip of my tongue to the bottom of my upper lip. I'd draw out the *L* sound. Lllll. ChaLLenge."

"Change."

"Look at me. ChaLLenge. Two Ls in the middle," I said. "Le, le, le."

"ChaLLenge," she said. "Le, le, le."

"A call or summons to engage in any contest," I said.

The card with that definition was in the opposite row. "Do you see it?"

Jillian scrunched up her face in concentration so that her brow furrowed and her nose assumed the shape of a rabbit's. "No," she said.

"Look closer." I repeated the definition, slower this time.

Jillian scanned the list. "What was the 'denition' again?"

"It's deFInition, Jills. There's an *FI* in the middle."

More face scrunching. It was never Jillian who became impatient or discouraged. That was my job. "De-FI-nition," she echoed. "That one." She pointed to a card.

"Great job!" I said.

"Thanks, Daddy-O," she said.

And so it would go. When Jillian matched a pair correctly,

she'd remove it from the table. On the good nights, the words were pronounced and defined and the 16 cards were off the table in two hours. Eight vocabulary words, two hours. Fifteen minutes a word. The lifting was heavy and exhausting, on the good nights.

On the bad nights, it was something else. Jillian's lesser intellect intersected with her teachers' occasional apathy to produce in me a frustration that could slip into sadness. On nights when the homework careened off track, I could lose touch with Jillian's guts and determination. I'd fall down the rabbit hole and into despair.

"I can't find my 'signment book," Jillian said. That's how a bad night might start.

Dinner was finished and the table was cleared. Kelly was in the basement listening to music, and Kerry was taking a bath. Jillian and Dad were at the kitchen table, Jillian's books piled like dirty dishes, pencil box open, spiral notebook. "Where do you think your AS-signment book is?" I asked. I knew where this was going. It was now 7:30 p.m. It was going until 11:00 p.m.

"I don't know," Jillian said.

"Jillian. It is your responsibility to keep track of your as-signment book. You're in fourth grade. You're not a baby."

"I thought I had it."

"That doesn't help me. Find your AS-signment book," I said. At this point, I wasn't emphasizing the first syllable to help her pronounce the word. I was just doing it to goad her. I was doing it to vent my spleen.

Which was ridiculous, of course. We never wondered if Jillian cared as much about her work as we did. She cared more.

On nights it didn't go well, she'd apologize. "I sorry I let you guys down," she'd say.

"You didn't let us down" was our response. We owed it to Jillian to work as hard as she did.

We never mentioned grades with her, either. We didn't want her to feel any added pressure, beyond what she put on herself. Still, Jillian knew the difference between an A and a D. On the days she'd empty her backpack and a *D* paper fluttered out, she would lower her gaze. "I try my hardest," she'd say.

"That's all that matters," we'd answer. "You do your best, we'll do the rest."

Jillian's conscience doubled at homework time. She knew she had to put in the effort. She wanted to please. In the face of her desire to do well, my short fuse looked petty and childish. Lots of nights during homework, I wondered which of us had the syndrome.

"I got it!" Jillian said. She smiled. The assignment book was in the bottom-most canyon of the cavernous backpack, beneath a prehistoric sandwich.

"Okay. Whaddaya got?" I asked.

She had math problems, science questions and spelling words. But when we looked on the page Jillian had written down for the math problems, they weren't there. Problems 1-12, page 28, she wrote. There were no problems on page 28. None at all.

In ensuing years, we would include in Jillian's IEP a request that someone check her assignment book at the end of the school day to make sure it was accurate. We'd also demand that the homework be modified to match Jillian's ability. But this was fourth grade, and on the days Mary left it up to Jillian to get the assignments, we'd often resort to guessing.

"Jills, there are no problems on page 28," I said.

"Oh."

"What page do you think they're on?"

"I'm not pretty sure," Jillian said.

"How do you expect me to help with homework if you don't write down the assignments correctly?"

"I don't know, I guess," Jillian said.

"You don't know," I said. "I guess I don't either. So what do we do now, Jillian?"

Even a fourth-grader with a learning disability knew better than to offer another "I don't know."

"Look on another page," said Jillian.

ON NIGHTS SUCH AS this—when divining the assignment became as laborious as actually doing it—I would wonder about our mission to keep Jillian in a regular classroom. "Maybe she can't do it, Ker'," I'd say.

I wondered if we'd made enemies at school for no reason. Maybe their time-honored practicality was wiser than our insistent optimism, and we'd set up a target out of our range. Worse, we'd tried to make our daughter fit our definition of what a "free and appropriate" education should be. What constitutes "appropriate" when we can't even figure out the homework assignment?

"Some nights I think the school is right," I'd say. We'd be lying in bed. The house was dark and quiet, both kids were asleep in their rooms down the hall. This is when we did most of our deep discussing. "What if we're expecting too much?" I asked.

What if we were preparing Jillian for the wrong things? We'd assumed she'd get the classroom education given every other child. We believed she would learn like everyone learned, only more slowly. With peer modeling and social interaction, she'd achieve her potential, whatever that might be, far more easily than if she were segregated part of the day from her typical classmates.

What if meeting Jillian's potential didn't involve a traditional classroom education?

There were programs already in place for kids with learning disabilities. These were essentially vocational programs, where she could learn a skill that could lead to a paying job. Maybe that was the way to go. "I want to do what's right by Jillian, not what we believe she should have," I'd say.

What if Daniel Boone has missed the blaze on the tree? Were we taking the wrong trail?

Who's this for? Does Jillian want this? Or do we? She was a well-adjusted kid. Jillian could be happy assembling cardboard boxes in a sheltered workshop. Things that matter so much to the rest of us—money, status, appearances—were not issues in her world.

Kerry didn't agree. She was convinced that Jillian would rebel if she were simply in a vocational program. "I can see her in that environment, looking around at everything and being insulted."

I don't know. Part of Jillian's disability—part of her Down

syndrome-ness—is a lack of reflection. Jillian doesn't dwell on anything other than the here and now. That also means she's not at all self-absorbed.

"What if we're doing all of this for us?" I asked Kerry again.

This was my despair talking. Kerry, as usual, had the right answers. Jillian hadn't inherited her spirit from me. "It's not about whether she can do it," Kerry would say. "It's about giving her the chance."

Kerry reminded me that there were other children in Jillian's class who were not gifted academically, whose talents ran away from college and toward a trade. The difference was that the school allowed those kids to define their course. "We are not going to let the school tell us who Jillian can be," Kerry said.

She reminded me of our mantras: "Expect Don't Accept." And my favorite: "All we can do is all we can do."

I needed that speech every so often.

JILLIAN AND I FLIPPED through the math book, looking for problems 1–12 that were not on page 28. We found 12 problems on a page nearby, and the next afternoon, when she brought the homework back home, checked or graded, we'd find out if we'd guessed right. For now, we soldiered on.

Jillian learned math visually. She had small, round counters to shift, from the ones pile to the tens pile. She had a number line. She had her fingers. Math was labor intensive, but not difficult. At least not in fourth grade.

Once we had the math problems solved, we moved to spelling. Eight words, same as vocabulary, written on three-by-five cards.

"Store," I said.

We'd look at the card together. Nancy Croskey, Mary Smethurst, and other teachers in previous years had done a good job giving Jillian the building blocks for learning to spell. One of those was the concept of blends: Consonants that often appear together at the beginning of a word. Such as S and T. She'd also been taught vowel sounds, long and short, and that occasionally at the end of a word, E's would have no sound.

"Store."

"S-O . . ."

"Remember the blend."

"S-O . . ."

"Jillian," I said. I made the sound of the S-T blend. *Ssss-tuh.*

"S-T . . ."

The O threw her, because it didn't sound the way a typical short or long O sounded. "S-T-A . . ."

"Nope. Listen to me," I said. *"Aw.* What sounds like *Or?"*

"A . . ."

"No. Not A. What else?"

"E . . ."

"No, Jills. E sounds like *Eeee* or *Ehhh.* What else?"

She paused a few seconds. There came a point during every homework session when her determination would overtake my patience. Usually it wouldn't take long. Her will was built for the long haul. My patience ran a hundred meters. Because she was nothing if not sensitive and eternally trying to please— and a little afraid of the impending eruption of Mount Dad— she considered her next response carefully.

"O?"

"Yesss!" I sounded like Marv Albert, announcing a New York Knicks game. I threw my arms into the air. "*S-T-O . . .*"

Jillian said, "*S-T-O.*"

I made the *R* sound, my tongue tapping the roof of my mouth. "*Rrrrr. S-T-O-Rrrrr . . .*"

"*S-R,*" Jillian said.

"Okay," I said. "Let's try it again. *Ssss-tuh.*"

"*Ssss-tuh,*" Jillian repeated.

"*Aw,*" I said.

"*Aw.*"

"*Ssss-tuh . . . aw . . . Rrrrr.*"

"*S-T-O-R?*" Jillian asked.

"Yesss!" I about roared. "Now, spell 'store.'"

"*S-T-O-R,*" Jillian said.

So close. No time for frustration yet. That'd be like jogging the last ten meters.

"What letter did we say was sometimes silent?" I asked.

"*E?*" Jillian asked, hesitantly. She knew we were close, too.

"Yep. Now spell store."

"*S-T-O-E-R,*" Jillian exclaimed, pleasure making her face a moonbeam.

"Not quite, sweetie. Remember how we said that the silent *E* was usually at the end?"

She did.

"Okay. Then just put the *E* at the end," I said.

"*S-T-O-R-E,*" Jillian announced.

I burst from my chair. I raised my arms in the air and did a little man-dance around the kitchen, I chanted, "*S-T-O-R-E,* store, store, store!" I high-fived my brilliant, fourth-grade daughter who, after 20 minutes and countless repetitions, was now the owner of a brand new word.

Remember about the little wins?

Kelly had been able to spell "store" in kindergarten. We never quizzed him on how to spell "store." We simply assumed he could. But with Jillian, we relished her ability to spell "store."

I called Kerry down from her bath. "Spell 'store' for Mom," I said.

Jillian stretched it out for dramatic effect, like those kids in the National Spelling Bee. At least that's how I saw it. Maybe she was concentrating on every letter. That was more likely. No matter. "S . . . T . . . O . . . R . . . E," Jillian said.

Hugs all around. We weren't going to take this leap for granted. No sir. Jillian spelled "store" by gosh. Yes, she did.

And then . . .

"Again," Jillian said.

Again?

"Let's do it again."

And so we would. Every letter, every word. All eight words, until Jillian was perfect. Sometimes, it would take three hours. Three hours, to spell eight words. Eight high-fives, eight trips around the kitchen, eight reasons for joy. There we were at 11:00 p.m., dancing around the room.

The next morning at breakfast, Jillian would request that we go over the words again, one last time before the test. "I get one hundred percent," she'd say.

It went like this for about three years. The index cards, the blends, the vowel sounds. Don't forget the silent *E*. The hours in the kitchen, at the table, hope and fear and pride and dread.

Despondent wondering in the dark. Kerry lighting the candle. Jillian's forever ability to put one foot in front of the other, for as long as she needed to walk the trail. Kerry's better nature and patience. My well-intended wrath. The dancing.

Night after night after night. Homework was frustrating and exhilarating, triumphant and desperate. It was Jillian at her absolute, resolute finest, hauling her well-intended, sometimes fretful dad and her entirely on-board mom along for her ride.

Homework was the whole Down syndrome experience wrapped up in a single word.

CHAPTER 12

The Coffee Song

I like coffee
Coffee like me . . .
—PAUL

I dislike mornings. I favor evenings. Perky people irritate me. I am a sunset person. The day is done, the work has been put in. Time to sit back and assess, preferably with a beer and a cheap cigar. I've taken sunset photos all over the world, from the Parthenon to the Gulf Coast of Florida to Sydney, Australia. I achieve, then I reflect. I'd rather reflect.

Jillian, being Jillian, would rather achieve. Each school day, she sprang to life like a toy with new batteries. I stumbled down the stairs. We were the oddest of partners.

One school morning in her sixth grade of learning, she wondered, "Dad, why you not a morning person?"

I ask her not to speak to me.

"I a big morning person," she said.

Well, of course. Blasting from the womb in five minutes flat, I guess you would be. "Eat your Frosted Flakes," I said.

Kerry had left for school earlier, and Kelly had his own routine. By 7:00 a.m., both were out of the house. It was up to me to get Jillian ready for the bus. Most days, it was bearable. But if I'd been up late covering a game, it was something less. I was as functional as a bowlful of peas.

"Whatchoo doing today, Daddy-O?"

Huh?

"Are you working today, sports person?"

"Yes, as a matter of fact, I am writing today."

"'Bout what?"

"I dunno yet. Eat. You have five minutes."

"I have a spelling test today."

"Congratulations."

"I go get an A."

"That'd be great. Three minutes."

"I be ready," she says. "I always ready."

That was true.

Jillian was six years old and starting first grade the first time I walked her to the school bus stop at the end of the common drive. I held her hand as we walked, and thus began a ritual that would last for three years. Jillian was so small, she had to crawl up the bus steps. She looked like a climber, scrambling the last few feet up El Capitan. A year or so later, she did the same thing. I couldn't figure out why. She'd grown, in height and coordination. Why the crawl up the bus steps? I found out after school, when Jillian's teacher sent home a note wondering why someone had dressed her with both feet in the same leg of her culottes.

When Jillian was in fourth grade, she decided handholding was out. Well, okay. We still walked down together, though, a morning glory that never failed to amuse and enlighten.

"What are you going to learn today?" I'd ask.

"Everything," she'd say.

By sixth grade, Jillian was setting her alarm, making her bed and dressing herself. I'd stopped the gentle wake-up nudges the previous year. I missed them. They seemed the natural evolution from our evening dances around the family room. I never had to wake her or tell her how late she was. Sometimes, she had to wake me. By the time she got to intermediate school, fifth grade, she didn't need my help. I might as well have been furniture.

Jillian and I were partners at sunrise, committing conversation at the breakfast table. I didn't arise at dawn for her benefit. I took comfort in the ritual sameness, even as it evolved and I began to matter less. You never know how the bonding will occur with your children. You can't arrange it. It's the spontaneous product of the everyday. With Jillian and me, it was weekday mornings, across the table.

I'd quiz her on the homework from the night before. "Who lives in the White House?"

"George Washington."

"No. I mean now."

"George Bush."

I'd make sure the shirt she was wearing matched the shorts. For a while, I tied her shoes. I made her breakfast. Cereal and toast. I packed her lunch.

"No carrots," Jillian might say.

"They're good for you."

"They're not good. I don't like carrots."

"No," I'd say. "I don't mean they taste good. Even though they do. They're good for you. They're healthy."

Jillian had occasional trouble with the subtleties of the language. She was very literal.

"I don't like healthy."

Jillian usually complained about something. Just because you have Down syndrome doesn't mean you don't eat like a typical kid. I'd pack the carrots in a plastic bag, next to a peanut butter and jelly sandwich in a plastic bag, next to a pudding cup in a plastic container, next to a plastic spoon, in a paper sack. Heaven help the earth.

"You better eat those carrots," I'd say.

I'd ask her about her friends. "Katie be mean to me," she'd say.

Katie Daly was Jillian's best friend. Why?

"I not sure," she says. "She says she not going to sit with me for lunch."

"I'm sure you guys will work it out."

I invented a jingle about my morning cup of coffee. I called it, believe it or not, "The Coffee Song." It was brilliant:

> *I like coffee*
> *Coffee like me*
> *I don't like tea*
> *Make-a-me pee*

This never failed to get a giggle from Jillian, who was never too cool to manage a laugh at the strange things her father did. "Sing the Coffee Song, Dad," she'd say nearly every morning.

I invented new verses, equally memorable:

I like coffee
It's my favorite drink
It doesn't stink
Like N-Sync

"N-Sync doesn't stink," Jillian protested.

I'd announce a new rendition of the Coffee Song by tapping my spoon on the side of my cup. At which point Jillian would either leave the room or giggle, depending on her mood and tolerance level that day.

Tap-tap-tap-tap.

I like coffee
And ya should, too
It's my favorite brew
Doodle-dee-doo

This was the daily dialogue of our lives. For 15 or 20 minutes, 5 days a week, 10 months a year, Jillian and I paused long enough to solve the world's problems. I never did this with Kelly; he didn't need the sort of morning direction I believed his sister did. He'd hurtle down the stairs like a cattle stampede, slam a Pop-Tart into the toaster, give it all of 30 seconds and be out the door, not so much as a "See Ya" in his wake.

"Go to school," I'd mumble. "Learn something."

Jillian Time was slower. It allowed for discovery.

"Who are you eating lunch with these days?" I'd ask.

"My friends."

We might have heard from one of her teachers that Jillian was eating lunch alone. Her gregariousness kept her popular among her peers, but her disability could keep them distant. By the time Jillian reached intermediate school, the other kids were becoming arm's-length friendly. We worried that Jillian was lonely.

"What friends?" I'd ask.

Jillian would reel off half a dozen names. Well, okay.

"Everything good at school?"

"I love my school."

We'd leave the house for the bus stop, where we'd be joined by other kids from the neighborhood and their moms. Where we lived, everyone seemed to have children about the same age. Loveland was Mayfield, but without June Cleaver's pearls. Five or six kids from our block would be waiting for the bus at the same time. We parents would drink coffee and converse until it came. Just me and the other moms.

On the morning of her first day of sixth grade, it occurred to Jillian that walking with her father to the bus stop was no longer cool. It had occurred to me earlier than that, but being a selfish dolt, I waited for Jillian to bring it up. Jillian, being Jillian, resisted as long as she could.

She broached the subject at breakfast. "Dad, we need talk 'bout something."

"Okay."

"You know how I always be your little girl?"

Uh-oh.

Every time Jillian achieved some new bit of independence, whether it was tying her shoes or dressing herself or roaming the wilds of the neighborhood unassisted, she would suggest that she wouldn't always be my little girl. My reply always had something to do with even if she became the king of England, she'd still be my little girl.

"Yes, Jills. You will always be my little girl."

"Well, your little girl is growing up."

"I know."

"I don't want to hurt your feelings," she said.

"You won't. What's up?"

"Well, I in sixth grade now."

"Yes. Very proud of you."

"I know you like to walk to the bus stop with me, and I like it, too," she said. "I know you're my best father, and you're in my heart." Her lip started to bounce. Maybe mine did, too. "I know you love me, Dad, but I have to say something."

Okay.

"I think I want to go to the bus stop by myself now."

She was a big girl, she said, almost 13 years old. Maybe it was "not 'propriate" that a dad be seen at the bus stop with his entering-sixth-grade, almost-teenaged daughter.

After I took a second to digest the new vocabulary— "Jillian, you said 'appropriate,' that's awesome"—I agreed that, sigh, a father doesn't need to be walking his blooming teenager to the school bus stop.

The first day I didn't walk her to the bus stop was the most melancholy of days. Mortality hit me like a brick. After years of it, I should have been a pro, accustomed to the ritual of her leaving home and coming back. It should have been a comforting era of "Have-a-Good-Day," followed later by "How-Was-Your-Day." My kids left every day, but they always came back.

But I wasn't a pro, and I never got used to it. Every year

was a little harder. My melancholia danced in lockstep with my advancing years. Overnight, I'd go from school's out and a houseful of people around me to the deafening silence of nothing but the dog at my feet. That first day of school was always the ultimate evidence that things would never be the same.

As a sports writer, I've written lots of swan songs for retiring athletes, some graceful, all sad. Each time I do one, I'm struck with the notion that the reader and I are grieving more for ourselves than for the subject of the story. We are remembering when. We were younger then. I watched Jack Nicklaus win the Masters at age 46. He seemed impossibly old at the time. As I write this, I am ten months short of my 55th birthday.

On this latest first day of school, Jillian is 12 years old, almost 13. It's a half-here, half-there age, too old for dolls and Disney, yet too young for makeup. On the cusp of . . . something.

"Sixth grade, Dad," she says. "I almost a teenager."

"Don't remind me," I say.

I brush her hair. The radio is on. Bob Dylan is singing "Just Like a Woman." Something about ribbons and bows. Dylan wasn't talking about the first day of school or how the separation was again going to slay the father of a daughter on the cusp. At least, I didn't think he was. But that's how I took it.

Tap-tap-tap-tap.

"Wanna hear the Coffee Song?" I suggest lamely.

"Da-a-a-d."

Each year, the spool unravels a little more, extending the distance between Jillian and me. She isn't my little girl anymore—even though she will always be my little girl. I get my game face on.

Jillian doesn't know it. But I worry about the ribbons and the bows. I always worry about the ribbons and the bows. "C'mon, sweets," I say. She has gotten dressed and finished her breakfast. She puts the finishing touches on tying her shoes. I send her to the door. Jillian runs alone to the corner to wait for the bus to take her to her first day of sixth grade. It was raining a fine mist. I thought that was 'propriate.

"Have a good day, Dad," Jillian yelled back at me.

Father Time is a thief. He gets better at his work as the years accumulate. Sixth grade becomes seventh, and I am with Jillian at the father-daughter dance, spiraling around a middle school cafeteria. Hopeless again, in the grip of melancholia or wonder, or whatever sort of love makes you want to laugh and cry at the same time. She is wearing a dress. I'm in a sport coat and slacks. "We're a lovely couple," Jillian observes.

It was just last week, I'm sure of it, that six-pound Jillian and I toured the family room to the simple poignancy of "Goodnight, My Love."

In a few years, she will extend the separation. By high school, she'd ride with Kerry. She'd get her own breakfast in the helter-skelter way her brother had. She won't need me. I'll pretend to be asleep as I hear the opening of the garage door. Usually, I'll get up right after Kerry and Jillian leave. After a summer of full throats, the house became perfectly silent and brooding, a fine stage for my proud sadness. The letting go was tough for all of our kids. It was tougher with this kid.

We measure our mortality in any number of ways: The never-before pain in the lower back after a day hauling mulch around the yard. The time it takes to fall asleep. The things we can no longer recall. We used to find our car and lose our keys. Now, we lose both. Life starts to hold more past than future. Even as we do our best to look ahead.

And now my little girl wouldn't be holding my hand.

"Have a good day," Jillian yells back to me, on the first day of sixth grade.

"Okay. I will," I say. "You have a great day, too." Jillian doesn't hear the last part. She's off to the corner, to catch the bus without me.

Bye, sweetie. See you this afternoon.

In the new version of the movie *Father of the Bride,* Steve Martin lies in bed awake the night before his daughter Annie's wedding. A montage of Annie moments follows: Annie as a baby, Annie riding a bike, wearing braces, playing basketball in the driveway. Annie sliding down the banister, wearing her high school cap and gown. Annie with her fiancé.

The scene lasts maybe a minute. Nowadays, I see Jillian's life that way too. A highlight reel. Two decades in sixty seconds. Soon enough, she'll be dancing at her high school graduation: Seals and Crofts singing "We May Never Pass This Way Again." I'll be standing speechless at the beauty and lightspeed of it all. A familiar well of entirely conflicting emotions will take hold, and I will be walking again in the rain, through the sunshine.

"That's the thing about life," Steve Martin says in the movie. "The surprises. The little things that sneak up on you and grab a hold of you." He continues: "I remember you were four. You had a red ribbon tied in your hair."

I remember that, too. All fathers remember. It's what guides us and propels us, even as we wish we could slow down, stop, rewind. Just for a day. You can't know where you're going without understanding where you've been. Today, I sing the Coffee Song. Tomorrow, I'll say, "Remember that?"

Tap-tap-tap-tap.

CHAPTER 13

The Two-Wheeler

Life is what happens to you while you're
busy making other plans.
—JOHN LENNON

We always had plans. There were tee-ball games to attend, homework to attempt, grass to be cut, the whole suburban catalog. Days, weeks, months passed, full and fulfilling. But rarely remembered. Whenever Kerry asked me what I wanted for Christmas, I said, "Time."

Time to linger, to savor, to remember why we came. To remember the little wins. If we're too busy to tend to those, we lose the foundation for our larger successes.

Jillian was 12 years old when she decided she would ride a two-wheeled bike. She saw other kids riding and assumed she would too.

"I do that," she said. Kelly was motoring down the drive, the pedals of his ten-speed bike whirring frantically.

"What?"

"I wide bike," she proclaimed.

This was a big step. We'd always allowed her to try everything. We wanted to keep with our belief that Jillian would do everything that every other kid did so we encouraged her to try bike riding as soon as she was able. But in keeping with her personality, Jillian decided she was ready for the two-wheeler before we'd had a chance to give it a lot of thought.

This was serious. This was a calamity in waiting.

"We'll see," I gulped.

" 'Bout what?" Jillian shot back.

"About riding a two-wheeler."

"I can do it, Dad."

That spring we bought Jillian a two-wheeler. It was comically small. The seat barely reached my knees. I am only five foot nine. It also had training wheels. That was a deal breaker: No training wheels, no two-wheeler.

"I don't need those," Jillian noted as I attached them to the bike frame.

"Oh yes you do, superstar," I said.

"I wanna wide like Kelly," she insisted.

"And you will. Just not right away." That seemed to satisfy her.

A considerable degree of balance and coordination is involved in keeping a human body aligned with the frame and skinny tires of a bicycle. So much so that riding a bike wasn't seen as entirely within the grasp of someone like Jillian. On the day she was born, we heard an impressive catalog of Down syndrome Can't Do's, and one I clearly remember was: "Jillian probably will never be able to ride a bicycle."

We didn't believe that, of course. We didn't spend all these years wheeling our daughter to this therapy and that to then deny her a chance to put it all into impressive play. If Jillian couldn't ride a big-girl bike, fair enough. She would get the chance.

We got her a helmet, the smallest we could find. It slid around her head like the tan skin of a white onion. Even after we pulled the chinstrap as tight as we could, the helmet wobbled. What were we getting ourselves into?

We started in early spring. Jillian had no problem pedaling the bike. Steering and turning took a while longer. So did getting off the bike. Jillian's first attempts at this meant stopping the bike and falling over.

The training wheels didn't always stay flat on the driveway, which caused the bike to shimmy, like the helmet. This wasn't all bad. It forced Jillian to use her gross motor skills for balance. It also alerted our fearless kid to the possibility that caution was not a bad option.

Not that she noticed much.

"I like this," Jillian decided. "I like this a lot."

As with most things, Jillian took a long time to master a two-wheeled bicycle. This provoked a few competing emotions: Frustration and impatience, at which I was already quite skilled. And lingering, a talent I'd lacked completely before Jillian's arrival, and only now was beginning to appreciate.

Twenty-first-century humans aren't good at lingering. Our moments don't build so much as simply appear and vanish, like a fence viewed from the window of a moving train. So much is lost in the motion.

I don't remember when Kelly first laughed, for example. I

try, but I can't recall when he tied his shoes or made his bed or managed a set of steps by putting one foot in front of the other. "What was Kelly's first word?" I asked Kerry, not long ago.

She didn't know, exactly. She thought it might have been "Deja." Deja-Vu was our shepherd-collie. But Kerry wasn't sure.

We might have made note the first time Kelly used a fork or spelled his name. It might have provoked a smile or a hug or a high five. Something worthy of the win. I don't know. We were always on to the next thing.

We did a lot of running in place, and it was exhausting at times. The suburban bargain can be one-sided if all you're doing is swimming manically to keep it afloat. Between tending to Jillian's unique needs, Kelly's typical wants, going to work and maintaining a house, the best Kerry and I managed most weekends was a rented movie and a pizza on Friday night before collapsing into bed.

Jillian slowed us down. We had no choice. All her firsts might have been seconds in our house: First steps, first words, first time going to the bathroom solo and diaper free. But because she was Jillian, we noticed. So much with her, we were told, would take longer. Just as much might never happen.

We preferred to see it as lingering over the Christmas presents, or a drive on what the author William Least Heat-Moon has called the "blue highways." Backroads traveling, on two-lane roads—the blue squiggles on a standard road map—gains in moments what it loses in hours. Jillian's progress wasn't the whoosh of a typical child's. It was a breeze through the screen-porch windows.

More than anything, the letting go of our bus-stop ritual

reminded me of the need to savor moments. So much of Jillian's life had made that point plain. Still, I tended to forget. Savoring is easy to say and hard to do. *Take the time. Make the time,* I told myself.

"Dad, come here quickly," she said to me one morning, not long after she turned ten. Getting over the initial pleasure-shock of Jillian's using the word "quickly," I got up from the breakfast table and found her in the family room. I watched as she tied her shoes for the first time.

Jillian took the strings to her sneakers, crossed them and pulled. She made two loops and crossed them, high enough in the loop to leave a hole underneath big enough to pull a loop through. Jillian nimbly stuffed one of the loops through the hole and pulled it tight. "See?" she asked.

It wouldn't have been an occasion if we hadn't been working on it for months. Every morning before school, Jillian would slip on her sneakers, then look at me. The look was her request: "Tie my shoes." And every morning, I would look at her and shake my head: "No. Do it yourself."

The tug-of-wills always ended when Jillian's dexterity didn't match her effort. I'd tie the shoes, the way her occupational therapist had instructed. I'd talk Jillian through it.

"Cross the laces like this, okay?" I'd say. She'd nod.

"Make the two loops, one for each lace. Cross them like this. Stuff one under the other and pull." Every day, she'd try. Every day, I'd finish. Every day, Jillian would get a little sadder but no less determined. And every day, I wondered when my beautiful, little ten-year-old girl would perform this simplest of routines.

It was this way with just about everything. Spelling to

shoelaces. With Jillian, you straightened your resolve and opened up a ten-pound can of patience. I'm not a fisherman, but I imagine fishing is similar to getting a 12-year-old Jillian to spell a two-syllable word. You have to enjoy the sunrise, not itch for the catch.

"I did it!" Jillian squealed with delight. "Just like a big girl."

Duly noted. You don't have to coax joy from the ordinary. You just have to invest in it.

Jillian went to school that day. She made her teacher watch her tie her shoes. She asked the teacher to stop class briefly so every kid in the class could watch her tie her shoes. "Listen up," Jillian announced. "I gonna do something here."

When Kerry got home that afternoon, Jillian was waiting in the kitchen. "Mom, I need to show you something," Jillian said. When Kelly got home, she repeated the performance.

She called both sets of grandparents. "I a big girl," she announced, still not so big, however, that she could include a verb in the declaration. Her rites of passage were no different from Kelly's, yet there was more to savor. The wonder was in the striving

She was 11 years old when she first wrote her name in cursive. Her J-I-L-L-I-A-N was curvy and swirling and took a full minute to achieve. She held the pencil so tightly, the tips of her fingers went white. "Now," she proclaimed immediately upon finishing, "time for Daugherty."

Six weeks into the bike experiment, Jillian announced, "Dad, time to take the t'aining wheels off."

"Not yet. You're not ready," I replied.

"When?"

"When you show me you're ready."

"Let's go," she said.

By late spring, I removed the training wheels. "There you go," I said.

Jillian was scared. Without the crutch of the added wheels, she became reluctant to test the common drive. Kerry and I had to force her, which was entirely unlike our child, who didn't usually need to be pushed into things.

"I don't know if I do it," she said to me one day.

"You won't know unless we try."

We started by helping her onto the bike and simply standing there with her. I'd straddle the front of the bike, a leg on either side of the front tire, keeping her perfectly upright. I held her around her waist. After a few days of that, I took my hands away and simply straddled the front tire.

"Sit straight up on your seat," I'd say. "Don't lean either way."

"I'm scared."

"Everybody's scared the first time they ride a bike," I said. "You'll be fine."

We graduated to me holding the back of the seat as Jillian offered those first tentative pushes of her legs on the pedals. "Don't let go," she said.

"I won't," I answered.

"Okay, Daddy-O. Let's go."

Jillian has never seen herself as disabled. She knows she has Down syndrome, but she doesn't believe she's different, if that makes sense. Her disability is more of a concept to her. She lacks the capability to take an intellectual accounting of who she is, and how she's different from her peers. It just doesn't occur to her. Or if it has, we've never heard her talk about it. We've never heard her say, "I wish I didn't have Down syndrome."

"Jillian doesn't even know she's short," Kerry has noted. And she is. She's four feet eight inches tall, and she has stopped growing.

At a party once, Jillian was making the rounds with a buddy of hers, who also has Down syndrome. "This is my friend Allison," Jillian said to everyone she and Allison met that day. "She has Down syndrome."

While she was learning to ride the bike, there were days when Jillian stood in the garage, helmet slippy, bike at the ready, and I knew she didn't want to do it. Maybe she'd fallen especially hard the day before. We'd gotten pads for her knees and elbows, ones like those worn by roller bladers. The padding was scuffed and driveway-stained after the first day.

"I a little bit nervous, a little bit," Jillian said.

"I know, sweetie. But you're getting better. It won't be long now."

We'd wheel the bike down the driveway, to the flatness of the common drive. I'd place both my hands on the back of the seat. She'd climb into the saddle and start pedaling. I'd jog lightly behind her. She'd ask if I had her. I'd assure her I did.

It went this way for a few weeks. Whenever I'd let go completely, Jillian would turn the wheel abruptly and without reason, fall over and scrunch up her face, auditioning a cry. Sometimes we'd quit at that point. But not often.

"Let's go," she'd say.

Kelly had figured out his two-wheeler in one afternoon. He might have had training wheels. I don't recall. He mastered it in a few hours. Maybe that's why I don't have the slightest memory of it. What was the day like? Cloudy, sunny, or cool? How old was he? What was the look on his face? What look did I have on my face?

I remember what it felt like when my father first let me go. It was a whoosh of freedom. It was weightless elation. I'd escaped some earthly shackle even as the tires were in complete connection with the road. I'll always remember it.

Did Kelly feel the same?

I don't remember if I even asked him.

Learning to ride a two-wheeler is a landmark experience in a kid's life, but without the struggle, it's an assumed act. It's special, without being special. That describes so much of typical childhood.

I let Jillian go a few fingers at a time. Ten fingers gave way to eight. Two thumbs gripping the top of the seat back were loosed. "You have me?" Jillian would ask, halfway down the drive.

"Yes."

Something occurred during those sessions with the bike. Time slowed, so memory could keep up. The more we practiced, the finer the clarity of the recollection became. Imagine printing a photograph in a darkroom. You dropped the photo paper into the developing solution, then swished it around the bottom of the pan. The image appeared, though it was hazy at first. The longer you swished, the richer the detail got.

I remember the day Jillian conquered the bike. It was blue-perfect, page one in the spring catalog of days. A small wind was blowing, nothing serious enough to alter the course of the bike; it was just warm enough to remind us summer was on its way. Ten fingers on the seat became eight. That became four—index and middle fingers, asserting minor control on the navigation system. Four fingers became two. Barely holding on now . . . holding on the way a fork holds soup.

"You have me?" Jillian wanted to know.

I said yeah. Then I didn't.

Jillian was 20 yards down the drive before she realized she was alone. "I wide!" she proclaimed.

I remember that. It was more than a decade ago, but I can summon it easily. Shiny copper, freshly minted on the new penny of recollection.

It's a moment I lean on now. I'll be on the golf course late in the day, and I will notice the particular slant of dusk as it leans over a fairway in June before settling like a quilt over the greenness. I will take in the warmth and the solitude and the softness. On an especially cold and bruised day in January, I will close my eyes and fetch that sunset memory. I will make it do my bidding.

Ordinary blessings are noted and recalled. The out-of-the-blue phone call from Kelly, now working in Brooklyn, a 12-hour drive away. The airy warmth of Kerry's fingers on the back of my neck, and the solitude of our local park, on the hyper-blue day after a winter ice storm. The spot in the center of our golden retriever's back, where the itch is perpetual, and she can't reach it. I get down on my knees, she hops up. I place her front paws squarely on my shoulders. I scratch the itch she can't reach.

Bruce Springsteen once sang about it not being a sin to be glad to be alive.

Jillian pedaled down the drive and away. "Dad," she announced. "I doing it!"

She'd moved the stars and the sky. I was there to bear witness. And to recall. To recall.

The Little Miami Bike Trail is a wonderfully maintained path a few miles from our house. It is straight and level and blacktopped. It follows an old railroad route along the meander of the Little Miami River for 75 miles, from Cincinnati almost to the state capital in Columbus. In certain spots where the trail bisects a small town, traffic can be heavy. Mostly, it's open road through farmland. It's a great place for a kid to stretch her wings and fly on her two-wheeler. The last time we rode, Jillian and I did 25 miles on that trail.

Not bad for a child who wasn't supposed to be able to ride a two-wheeler. Better for her ancient dad, who gets to savor the ride twice. In person and in memory.

CHAPTER 14

Sometimes

Regrets, I've had a few
But then again, too few to mention.
—PAUL ANKA

Helping Jillian master the bicycle was like planting a prayer flag atop Mount Everest. Other times, the effort simply wore us out. Raising a child with a disability can be like eating at a five-star restaurant and having someone pick your food for you. The experience will be good but not what you expected.

Sometimes, I wish Jillian were a typical child.

It is a selfish wish, confined to its own atoll by the daily joy Jillian brings. But it's there, nonetheless, even as I wish it would go away. I love Jillian with a part of me no one can touch. It's a deeper chamber, protected by its own moats and deadbolts. That place can't be diminished or compromised. But the limitations imposed by Jillian's needs are never fully reconciled.

A framed photograph hangs on the wall of my office at home. Called "Hartwig House, Truro," it was taken in 1976 by a well-known professional named Joel Meyerowitz. It looks down a first-floor hallway to the screened front door of an older home on Cape Cod, Massachusetts. The hallway walls are covered in thick white paint, generations of coats. The floor is wide-planked hardwood, painted a grayish blue. I'm thinking that by now, a new owner might have sanded away the dull floor paint to reveal the scars and heaves of the original floor.

The two throw rugs, white with floral stitching, rectangular and faded, dress up the gray-blue.

This is a sturdy house, a house of generations leaving but always coming back, dutiful fathers and mothers and respectful children, catching fireflies in Mason jars at dusk. Enjoying.

The photograph shows a bedroom, barely. It appears on the far right, offering a sliver of a glimpse inside. We see part of a bed and a wooden dresser, above which hangs what looks to be a black-and-white wedding picture. The groom appears to be about to remove the bride's garter, but it's hard to tell. The bedroom is mysterious but incidental.

It's a clear day, probably early in June. It's late morning. Soft sunlight colors the hallway walls and floor. Not yet the garish glare of midday. This is what I'm guessing as I stare into the picture.

Directly down the hall is the wooden front door, heavy and permanent, half open to a screen door, beyond which are teases of green. The photo is an invitation to come into the daylight. Explore, seek, wander. It is a new day, a summer day, full of its own mysteries, yielding its own endless possibilities.

Walk down the hall, past the bedroom on the right and the

suggestively half-open front door. Push open the screen door. Escape.

That's what I think of whenever I stare at that photo on the wall of the office in my house. Escape. If I stare at it long and hard enough, I can will myself into that summer day.

Expanding Jillian's dreams means constricting our own. This isn't a complaint. It's not bitterness. It's just a fact. Her goals tug at ours. They are not compatible. Our lives are less separable than the lives of typical parents and their grown children.

Sometimes, I resent that.

Centuries and generations ago, homes were multigenerational. Economics demanded it. So did a lack of easy mobility. Children became adults in the same place where they grew up because they couldn't afford to get away. That's happening again now as the economy continues to lurch. But it is the exception.

Most parents tote the world for 18 or 22 years, maybe a little longer depending on how many children they have. Then, they heave that refrigerator off their backs and begin seeing the world instead of lifting it. How they define that world is up to them: Hawaii, Europe, Atlantic City, a mortgage-burning party.

After a finite amount of time they are paroled.

We will never be paroled.

Kerry and I celebrate Jillian's milestones. We rejoice when she is 14 years old, in seventh grade, in a regular-ed classroom, fully included. She rides a two-wheeler, she makes her bed. She is respected at school, if not always befriended. Our combined efforts have been entirely worthwhile. Rewarded and rewarding. And yet, the effort needed to get Jillian to where she is now has come at the cost of pursuing our own interests. We have gained much in helping Jillian to the life she has. What we've lost—and will continue to lose—is time to explore our own lives.

Our best friends are the parents of Jillian's friends. Our social life revolves around Jillian's needs, social and otherwise. This is unusual only in the number of years we will have to do it. All parents sacrifice for their children, whether it's escorting them on dates or taking a second job to pay for college. But in homes with typical children, that responsibility comes with a shelf life. Ours is open ended.

I want to retire somewhere south of Ohio. Winter in this state can be a time for reflection and solitude and the beauty of fresh snow on a fallow field. It can also be gray, depressing and a reason to move. In Ohio, it gets to 35 degrees and cloudy sometime after Thanksgiving, and stays there until the first of March. This is three-plus months of wondering what we're doing here considering that we are people of free will.

I dream of South Carolina. I picture short winters and long days on the golf course. There is no snow shovel in my dream—nor is there a car that has quit for lack of a battery spark. There are long, cool drinks on the deck out back and short days of fulfilling, semi-retired labor. Being retired is something to which I aspire easily.

It won't happen.

We won't leave the social network Jillian has established in Cincinnati. I won't retire, at least not completely, until I am forced to. I will have to allow for myself and Kerry, and also for Jillian, for as long as I am able. Jillian will work. It might even be full-time work. She will earn a living. But it probably won't be enough for her to live on.

Jillian won't have children. Kerry and I will be grandparents only if Kelly has kids.

I realize all this. I accept it. But when I study it and dwell on it, I look at that photo of that house in Truro, Massachusetts, on that fine summer morning of infinite promise, and I feel cheated.

I read Karl Taro Greenfeld's book *Boy Alone* not long ago. It is the story of a family's game attempt at dealing with a mentally challenged son. It takes place the 1970s, and Noah Greenfeld is profoundly autistic. Karl is Noah's brother. The way Karl Greenfeld describes it, his family is held captive to this child who is incapable of responding to even the simplest gestures of human communion. Noah avoids eye contact. He smiles at odd times. He rocks on the floor, and he manipulates rubber bands with his fingers.

Karl wonders, how do you love someone who doesn't love you back? At what point does love harden into obligation? Your heart never leaves the equation, not entirely. It recedes, from the pounding it takes. You never stop trying, even when you stop believing.

Karl's father writes of the strain Noah's disability puts on his marriage: "How can we have faith in a marriage that has biologically backfired?" In *Life* magazine in 1970, Josh Greenfeld writes, "Until I had a child like Noah, I automatically believed in the institutions of organized medicine, private philanthropy and public programs. Where there's an ill, I naively thought, there must be a way. The school Noah has been attending does not have the operating capital to provide the mentally ill or mentally retarded child with the same full-time, one-on-one treatment therapy he so desperately needs."

Ultimately, the Greenfelds break. They assign Noah to a group home in Southern California. Noah is sent away for being Noah, like the family dog who bites the neighbor's kid. It doesn't work out. Noah is bruised and shows signs of sexual abuse so they bring him home. Eventually, when all the wells have been tapped and found dry, the family exiles Noah to save what's left of itself. Noah winds up in an institution. "Twice-imprisoned" is how Karl Greenfeld describes it. The father isn't so kind. Josh Greenfeld refers to his autistic son as "genetic rot."

Josh even consults the playwright Arthur Miller, who had a son with Down syndrome. Miller tells Josh Greenfeld, "I put him in a nursing home straight from the hospital. I had a Down syndrome cousin. Ruined the family. Brought the family down trying to care for him." Miller eventually moved his son to a state institution. "He's a healthy kid, and we visit him. But it's different. It's not as if we became attached to him." Trying to reach the unreachable boy, Karl Greenfeld alternates between caring deeply for his brother and discovering how deep his own well of resentment can be.

Beyond the ceaseless striving to always do what's best, there isn't much in *Boy Alone* that resonates with us. Jillian is communicative and all-loving. Her disability is far more receptive to whatever one might define as "treatment," most of which is opportunity and patience. There was never discussion of adoption when she was born. There is no talk of "group homes" now. Jillian has added immeasurably to all our lives. She gives more than she receives.

But to an extent, Jillian rules our days. And she always will. Disability puts a ring around your life. It is a moat that surrounds even those who can swim.

It's not terrible. It's not even burdensome, most of the time. It is annoying but not life-changing that Jillian will always need to be driven places, even as she masters public transit. It irritates when traffic backs up or I'm mad about something else.

What gets to me are the dream restrictions. Sometimes.

Kerry and I celebrated our 20th anniversary in 2003 with a week in a bungalow high in the hills of St. John, in the US Virgin Islands. A rutted, perpetually muddy road, negotiable only by four-wheel-drive vehicle and a multitude of resident goats, led to the one-room house we rented for a week. The views were spectacular: Thick forest canopy, sloping to crescents of sand. Water changing from green to blue and back, depending on its depth and the way the sunlight struck its surface. The place was a Caribbean postcard.

The house was in Coral Bay, at the far end of St. John, away from the cruise boats and the day-trippers over from St. Thomas, snorkels and underwater cameras in tow. At the base of our hill, by a small boat dock, was a restaurant: Skinny Legs. Calling this place a restaurant was generous. In 2003, it was an island dive, a roof, a bar, some stools and several four-top tables. Two guys originally from the States ran Skinny Legs. You could get cheeseburgers there, and Carib beer, and not much else.

I befriended one of the guys. Doug Sica lost his job as an electrician in New Jersey in 1978. He applied for 52 jobs, and the first offer he got was on St. John. He and his wife and two small kids moved from Jersey in August of that year. The job didn't start for four months. In the meantime, Sica tended bar. He tended bar for the next 12 years. Someone else took his electrician's job.

Sica had a friend already on the island when he arrived. Moe Chabuz was also a bartender, in Cruz Bay, the island's largest town. In 1991, the pair sold a boat they owned jointly and spent the proceeds on a ramshackle watering hole called Red Beards, at the other end of St. John, in Coral Bay.

They renamed the place Skinny Legs after Moe's pencil-legs. It opened in May of that year, and struggled. Opening a restaurant where most of your customers arrived by sailboat maybe was not a spotless idea. In 1991, Skinny Legs had no tables or food, only alcohol. "It took us nine months to save enough money to buy the grill and the [exhaust] fan," Sica told me. By the time Kerry and I visited 12 years later, Skinny Legs was alive with grill smoke and bottled beer.

Sica told me he didn't have bad days. "I don't allow them," he said. Living in paradise doesn't immunize one from bad days, but it can't hurt. Paradise doesn't come cheaply, though. Paradise takes guts. Sica took a big chance, and it made all the difference.

Doug Sica died two years after we spoke, at the age of 56. "After a short illness," according to the Skinny Legs website. Moe sold the place on April Fool's Day in 2012. But what a time they had.

I've told this story a hundred times. I get to the end, and I say, "One of these days." I admire people with the courage to take audacious leaps. I daydream about it. "One of these days . . ."

I won't though. I won't leap. One of these days is someone else's idyll.

Kerry and I do have a post-retirement bucket list. We want to go to Las Vegas on the first weekend of the NCAA basketball tournament, to spend hours in a casino sports book, making silly bets. We want to spend several months living in Ireland. We want to rent a villa in Tuscany. And we want to watch the Super Bowl at Skinny Legs. These are wonderful wishes, but they are fragments of a dream. What we want to do will always be harnessed to what we have to do.

Typical parents might say, "Let's move to Southern California and live in the sunshine every day." They might decide, after retiring, that Italy would be a pleasant place to spend a few years. Ireland works for me. We could do that—if Jillian agreed to come along.

Financially, Jillian limits us, too. There is government money, but not a lot. We want Jillian to be as independent as possible. The more money she earns, the less she'll get from the feds. That's as it should be. It's also another chain on our retirement. Helping Jillian more means helping ourselves less.

A few years ago, I was on an airplane, coming back from covering a Cincinnati Bengals game in Oakland. A woman sitting in the center seat of the row in front of me was looking at family pictures on her laptop computer. Snapshot after snapshot of healthy, smiling daughters, two of them, maybe ten and eight years old: Swimming in a backyard pool, at a costume party, posing with their mother and father. Perfect.

I gazed between the seats at the images. I was jealous. I resented this woman and her two beautiful, perfect kids and the smooth arc I imagined they'd follow through life.

These kids, this family: They have no idea. No IEP meetings for them. No constriction. No strangers noticing their kids' faces, the way some notice Jillian's, then looking away, into the safe middle distance. The taxi service stops at age 16 for those parents. The bank vault closes five or six years later.

After that horrible first night of Jillian's life, I stopped feeling as if I'd been robbed. It was pointless to feel cheated or guilty or ashamed. It dishonored the effort needed to build a better Jillian. As the months and years progressed, I even started to feel blessed to have fathered a child with a disability.

I know things that you do not. Jillian has taught me.

But I'm still selfish enough to look at this beautiful 13-year-old before me and see someone whose needs will take precedence over my own. It feels unfair.

A few hours after I got off the plane, after peering at the perfect little girls on the laptop screen, I came from the garage of my house and into my kitchen, where Jillian jumped into my arms and told me how much she missed me. I'd been gone barely 48 hours. "You're my best father," Jillian decided.

Life has its tradeoffs.

I don't think much about South Carolina anymore. Instead of dreaming of retirement, I pray I can stay employed in a choppy economy with little use for newspaper columnists. I get wishful though. That's when I stare at Joel Meyerowitz's photo. It is a late morning in early summer, sunny and bright and potentially momentous. The front door is open, the screen door awaits. I stare for a while. I imagine what that day must be like.

CHAPTER 15

Cymbidium Orchids Under the Porch Light

(Today I Met) The Boy I'm Gonna Marry.
—ELLIE GREENWICH, TONY POWERS,
PHILLIP SPECTOR

Jillian breezed through her days so effortlessly that we wondered sometimes what we weren't seeing. You hand your kids to strangers for six or seven hours a day, and you hope for the best. Until something dramatic occurs, you don't think much about it.

I didn't work in Jillian's classroom anymore. Intermediate school is a little advanced for that. We'd get the nightly 'signment book updates, attend the IEP meetings as needed. We'd listen to Jillian say her day was "great." We took it on faith, mostly. Part of me wanted to be at school, to see how Jillian was getting along. She wasn't shy, she was incurably positive. Jillian was easy to like. Who liked her?

You can't make the world see your kid the way you do. The random moments that told us who Jillian was, and who she could become, weren't often on public display. Just because we saw her as extraordinary didn't mean everyone else did. Every parent thinks his child is extraordinary.

We did well with things we could control. Jillian's education could be managed, even if it meant wielding the law like a cudgel. We could teach her social skills and basics such as counting money, ordering from a menu and, later, negotiating the byzantine public transportation system. We would give free rein to her will and her spirit. Mastering the bicycle was persistence exemplary enough to hang on a museum wall. There was never a problem allowing Jillian to be Jillian.

We couldn't make her peers be her friends, though. At a certain point, Jillian stopped getting invited to birthday parties and sleepovers. She ate alone in the school cafeteria. We couldn't do anything about that.

Perceptions can be changed. How kids choose their relationships is a little trickier. Jillian was fully included—but not in all things.

She never talked about the empty times at school. She didn't partly because she didn't believe there were any. No one was overtly cruel. If a peer had referred to her as a "retard" or something equally awful, Jillian would have been hurt. No one did that, ever. The separation was more subtle, and Jillian's mind wasn't locked into subtleties. She had plenty of room for compassion and empathy, but not much for introspection or acute observation.

If kids said "hi" to her, if they maintained a surface cordiality, that was enough.

We poked and prodded a little. Her answers were always the same:

"How was school?"

"Oh, I had a great time."

"What did you do?"

"Same stuff."

"What did you do at lunch? Sit with anyone?"

"Not really."

I never wanted to put it into Jillian's mind that sadness or self-pity could be a legitimate response to her occasional isolation. I never said, "Do you ever get lonely at school?" Instead, I'd ask of her solo lunch times, "Are you okay with that?"

"Yes, Dad. I fine."

I wondered what the other kids thought of Jillian. I imagined them liking her, in an arm's-length sort of way. Someone to say hello to, then move on. I put myself in their 12- or 13-year-old shoes. Would I be friends with Jillian? Would we hang out? Would the widening gap in her ability to communicate scare me away?

She looks different. How much does that matter?

I have no problem dealing with people with disabilities. I'm used to it. I'm an adult. What if I weren't?

When I was 10 or 11 years old, after my mother died and before my dad remarried, I spent the afternoons after school with my best friend. Mrs. McKee and Aunt Aline, who looked after me until my dad picked me up after work, lived on his street. The kids in the neighborhood spent lots of time playing sports in the street. One of them, a boy named Patrick, had Down syndrome.

On the infrequent afternoons when Patrick came outside, we included him in our games. Patrick wasn't as coordinated as the rest of us. He played with difficulty. When we played football, no one wanted to play center, so we assigned it to Patrick. We had no issues with him—he hiked the ball and blocked. But we didn't talk much to Patrick. I never found myself one-on-one with him, and I was glad about that. I didn't dislike him. He just made me uncomfortable.

We cheered when Patrick achieved things the rest of us did ordinarily. Nice block, Patrick. Way to hike the ball. It made us feel good about ourselves. When we finished our games, Patrick went home by himself. No one invited him to have a Coke. We didn't include him.

I look back at that time now with an informed regret. Feeling good and doing good aren't always the same. We patronized Patrick; we didn't befriend him. Sympathy without empathy can be hollow. If I met Patricks' parents now, I'd tell them I was sorry.

This isn't 1968, and Jillian isn't Patrick. But some of the same hesitations remain. That's how I perceived things with Jillian and her peers as she moved from elementary school to the intermediate building.

I wanted more for her than that. The seismic fun of childhood is a co-dependency. From the time she entered kindergarten, Jillian had willed herself into the mix. Socially fearless and engaging, Jillian wasn't left out until fourth or fifth grade when kids started to notice she was different. It was a constant tug. Each new achievement took Jillian closer to a life of independence and choices. Each advancing school season deepened the separation.

We'd gotten glimpses of Jillian's future. The Rutkousky girls next door outgrew her, one by one. First Elisabeth, the oldest and Jillian's age, then Jessie, a year younger. Finally, Anna, who was younger than Jillian by three years. Paths that once intersected on the common drive now diverged. It was the natural order of things.

"I go Jessie's house," Jillian said. It was a morning in summer, when Jillian was eight years old. She was up early, dressed and ready to rumble, before the rest of us had even pondered the day.

"I go Jessie's."

For a while, that was fine. Occasionally, Jessie would appear at our door, as Elisabeth had before her, and Anna would after. Jillian and Jessie would play. But after a few months, Jessie had other things to do. "But I love my Jess," Jillian would say, when we had to tell her Jessie was busy and couldn't play.

Months, even years, after Jessie had made it plain that she had other things going on, Jillian would spot her on the drive, and go tearing out of the house. "Jess, Jess!" she'd scream, delightedly. Jessie would get the best Jillian hug.

"Want come over my house?" Jillian would ask.

Kerry and I would intervene before it became too uncomfortable. "You need to give Jessie a little space," we'd say.

Kids grow, and the road forks. The Rutkousky girls were never anything but gracious. But their lives weren't Jillian's life.

Jillian was 12 years old when she last had a party that included typical kids. Ally Ballentine, a girl Jillian had been friends with since kindergarten, and Nancy Croskey's daughter Lauren came. They were polite. Twelve-year-olds are not practiced at the art of grin and bear it, though. It was the last time either was at our house.

Being in regular-ed classrooms didn't ensure a regular childhood. No amount of scholastic striving could overcome being excluded. Jillian's classmates were never mean to her. They just moved on. Jillian would make her way in the world. If she couldn't share the journey with friends and lovers, what would it mean?

I wanted her to experience the expectant glow of a porch light with a young man late in the evening. I wanted her to know the smell of his cologne. She had a right to experience the mysteries of attraction, shared under moonbeams with a boy who made her happy. Everyone has that right. This was my greatest hope. It was my deepest ache, too, because I couldn't do anything about it.

The possibility existed that some routine evening, Jillian would appear before us to announce she was different and want to know why. What would happen when the world stopped being her friend?

An image haunted me as Jillian passed through fourth grade to fifth, from the cocoon of elementary school to the multiple classrooms of intermediate school and beyond: A poster I'd seen, circa 1980, of a boy with Down syndrome. His head was bowed, his gaze ached. "I just want a friend," it had read.

One Friday night when Jillian was in sixth grade, as Kerry and I honored our exhaustion with a movie, a pizza and the couch, the poster came to life. Jillian entered the room crying.

"What's the matter, sweets?"

"I don't have any friends."

We told her that wasn't true. Actually, Jillian did have one very good friend. Katie Daly's family had moved to town three years earlier. Katie had Down syndrome. She was a year younger than Jillian, and they'd become inseparable. Still, hearing Jillian say she had no friends ached me in a deep and different place. There is no loneliness like the loneliness of a child.

Up to this time, we had owned a sort of reverse snobbery when it came to Jillian's social life. We had wanted so much for her to be fully included in school that we didn't put her in situations where she was associating with the kids in the special-education rooms. We wanted her role models and peers to be typical kids. Jillian went to tap class; she took ballet. Up to fourth grade, she played basketball and soccer with typical kids.

As she grew older, that left Jillian in an awkward and limiting place. She was too advanced socially—at least in our thinking—to be friends only with special-needs kids. Yet she was too far behind to hang with typical children. She was neither here nor there. Jillian's choices narrowed.

Kerry, who always had a better grasp on the actual, recognized that it was time to fix what she could fix. While I was dwelling on Jillian's fading bond with typical kids, Kerry marshaled the alternatives. "It wasn't a fear for me," Kerry said of Jillian's loss. "It was an inevitability."

She took the offensive, even while Jillian was still active with typical kids. When Jillian was in seventh grade, Kerry enrolled her in Special Olympics swimming and TOPSoccer, a program for kids with all manner of disabilities. The league's mission was straightforward: "To allow every child with special needs the opportunity to participate, contribute and excel in the game of soccer." Kids in wheelchairs played. Kids in walkers, kids on crutches. Autistic kids. Lots of kids with Down syndrome.

There was coaching and teaching. There were games and trophies and championships. Mostly, it was social. It was a chance for kids with disabilities to hang out. It was relaxed. Given the over-exuberance that rules youth sports now, it was nice. As someone who covers sports for a living, I thought the kids in TOPSoccer owned a perspective the rest of us should borrow.

It was also where Jillian met Ryan Mavriplis.

Ryan was two years older, and he attended a nearby public high school. He was every bit her equal, intellectually and socially. His parents had raised him the same way we'd raised Jillian. His mother, Ellen, would become so passionate about Ryan's education that she'd make it a career choice. The shingle hanging outside her office speaks to her philosophy:

Inclusion Advocates.

Jillian was about to turn 15 when she found herself alone with Ryan on the far corner of the practice field, acres from the eager ears of parents and teammates. It was her second year of TOPSoccer, and she'd known Ryan for more than a year. Ellen's husband, Dimitri, was her coach. Moms at practice had noticed their flirtations. Most thought nothing of it. Kids flirt all the time—even kids with disabilities.

"I would like to ask you something," Ryan began.

"What?" Jillian answered.

"Do you know that my school, Sycamore, has a Homecoming?" Ryan began.

"No."

"It's a dance. You go to dinner before. Have you ever been to a Homecoming?"

"No."

"Would you like to go with me to Sycamore's?"

Well.

I wasn't there when Jillian got that proposal. They both told us about it later. I wish I had been. Sunshine, in human form. I spent years fretting her social life. In one instant, all that vanished. My little girl would be going to Homecoming. Cymbidium orchids under the porch light.

Ryan approached the exalted moment with some trepidation. He was nervous. "I was afraid she might say no," he remembers

That was never a possibility. Jillian was at once happy and amazed. She pronounced Ryan "a gentleman." She began to blush: "You should have seen the expression on my face. I loved this guy."

"Love at first sight," Ryan says.

Kerry watched from a distance as Jillian and Ryan approached, beaming. Jillian was reserved for about a second. Then she smiled. Then she ran. "I have a date! I have a date!"

I'm not sure whom I wanted that moment for more. Jillian, of course. But for me too. Kerry and I had always been too busy advocating for Jillian to cry for her. I'd said to Kerry many times, "If Jillian isn't sad, we shouldn't be, either." Of course, I didn't believe that, even though Jillian was almost never sad. Kerry saw it differently. She had never doubted that Jillian would have boyfriends.

Jillian spent that night running around the house, offering

joy in a singsong voice: "I got a da-a-a-a-te! I got a da-a-a-a-te! Woohoo!"

She needed a dress. She needed shoes—open-toed, which meant she would need a pedicure. There is some sort of women's code that says no one can have a pedicure without also having a manicure. So Jillian would have that too.

She and Kerry spent an entire Saturday shopping for a dress. Fathers and sons play catch. Mothers and daughters hit the mall. They went to at least five stores, where Jillian tried on ten dresses. She loved them all. She couldn't stop looking at herself. Jillian's primary requirement was that the dress she chose be sheer enough to swoosh when she spun around. She spent an afternoon in dressing rooms, swooshing in lots of dresses.

They settled on a teal number that stopped just short of her knees. It had spaghetti straps. It sparkled.

Finding shoes was a challenge. Jillian's size-two feet were as tiny as she was. Short of buying a Barbie doll and stealing its high heels, the shoes had to be dressy, without looking like something a six-year-old would wear. They settled on a pair of black strapped shoes.

Kerry sewed Jillian a shawl to match the dress. On the day of the dance, she spent an hour doing Jillian's hair into a perfect mass of well-mannered braids and made sure her makeup was perfect. She applied the powder, the blush, the mascara and the lip gloss. Jillian liked the makeup. It allowed her to look at herself in the mirror, never a bad thing as far as she was concerned. It also gave her a reason to feel special in a way not always associated with kids like her. This wasn't just

Dad's dream being realized. Jillian beheld her reflection and found it pleasing.

"I beautiful, Mom," she said.

"Yes," Kerry answered. "You are."

Fifteen minutes away, Ryan Mavriplis was slipping into a suit and tie. He'd spent part of the day getting a haircut and a shave. He was 16 years old, a freshman in high school. I've often marveled since that night at the coincidences of great fortune that have filled Jillian's life. There have been so many of them that I don't find them coincidental anymore:

The amniocentesis that wasn't. The anger Jillian used in the hospital to help her breathe. Nancy Croskey, teaching fourth grade in our school district. And Ryan Mavriplis, being raised nearby, also to believe opportunity was a birthright.

He arrives at our house at 6:00 p.m. sharp. He is a young man in a black suit, white shirt, and a red tie. He strides purposefully up the sidewalk and to the door, offering me his hand. "Good evening, sir," he announces. "I am here to take your daughter to the Homecoming."

His parents, Dimitri and Ellen, stood just behind him, beaming, and followed Ryan inside.

We had no idea, then, what this evening would portend. It was just a first date. Lives are filled with first dates. Living with Jillian meant living in the moment. Anything else could be overwhelming. This was a fine moment.

Jillian stands at the top of the stairs, just out of Ryan's gaze. Her formal construction is complete: Dress and shawl, shoes and pedicure, manicure, braids, and makeup. I look up at her from the landing below. Ryan has moved on to more introductions, in the family room.

"Dad, I so nervous," Jillian says.

It's impossible to describe what she looked like in that instant. That's why we have poets and sunrises. Jillian was slim in her form-fitting aqua dress. Audaciously red lipstick propelled her into womanhood. She paused at the top of the stairs to catch her breath. She gathered her poise as she prepared to pass through this blooming window of time.

"Don't be nervous, sweetie" is what I manage to say. "It's going to be a great night. The best."

"Is Ryan handsome?" she asks.

"Yes, Jills. He is."

She begins a slow stride down the stairs and across some new and indefinable threshold. She holds the railing until she reaches my outstretched hand. "I so nervous," Jillian says again.

The day Jillian was born, I thought of this moment. I thought it would never occur, and I grieved. I pondered the cruelty of her best steps stolen, before she ever got to dance. Nearly 15 years earlier, to the day, I had hurt for my baby girl and what I believed would be a half full existence. A life without Homecomings and proms—and the promise of both—is no life at all. I wondered why God would do this to my daughter. Now, I am at the bottom of the stairs, holding her hand. Knowing that, in a few hours, she will dance.

"You look beautiful," I say.

In the years after this, as Homecomings, proms and anniversaries with Ryan assumed a familiarity, Jillian would wait downstairs and stare out the window until she saw Ryan's car turn onto the common drive. Then she'd run upstairs so Kerry could give her a proper entrance.

"In-tro-ducing . . . Miss Jillian . . . Phillips . . . Daugherty!"

She'd enter then, with all the poise and confidence of a runway model.

Not this time though. This was the first time, so she held my hand, maybe for the first time in the few years since she had asked that I not escort her to the bus stop.

"Ready?" I ask.

"Yes," she says.

Jillian takes the first walk of a lifetime then, down the hall and into the family room. Ryan waits, standing tall, a corsage box in his hand.

"Hey, Ryan," Jillian says.

"Hey, Jillian," Ryan says. "You look beautiful."

He removes the wrist corsage—an orchid!—from the box. "You want to put it on me?" Jillian asks. Ryan asks how. I help him get the corsage safely from the box. Kerry helps place the corsage on Jillian's wrist.

"That okay?" he asks.

The flower is on the underside of Jillian's wrist. She turns it upright. "Thanks, Ryan. You're so sweet. I got something for you, too."

Kerry takes Ryan's corsage from its box and pins it to the lapel of his suit.

Jillian says, "We're a good team."

They leave then, with Ellen and Dimitri, arm-in-arm across the lawn. We follow them to Ryan's house, where several of Ryan and Jillian's friends have gathered. Kids from soccer and

Special Olympics, mostly. They're all going to dinner first, and then the dance. Sparkling grape juice fills champagne flutes.

Ryan offers a toast: "I want to thank everyone for being here. To my good friends Ben and Robbie and Jacob and Margo and Jillian. I'm happy I have a date. Amen."

Jillian adds her own words: "I love this time to spend with my boyfriend. I love my coach. I love this very lovely evening. I really love you guys."

A year later, in the same spot, Ryan offered another tribute to the assembled revelers: "To my girlfriend I love with all my body and love I have in my heart. She's an angel and good at soccer and everything. Amen."

And amen.

Ellen swears now that in the backseat of the car, on the way to dinner that first night, Jillian said, "Ryan and me gonna get a 'partment and get married." We take Ellen's word on that one. None of us were that far along yet—at least not that night. The hope was there though that Jillian and Ryan would have such a chance.

They danced that night. "All the slow ones," Ryan said.

Jillian praised her boyfriend's dancing prowess: "Lots of good moves. I felt like I was in love."

I had worried Jillian's disability would come to define her. Then Ryan arrived. The door opened. Everything was possible again.

There have been nights, more than I could ever have imagined, when Jillian and Ryan have lived my dreams for her. They've lingered in the porch glow. The scent of cologne has become familiar. Ryan has felt the delicate touch of a young lady's fingertips on the back of his neck as they danced around the room. They have shared the mysteries. They've earned what lovers own.

That has all happened. But that first night, when Jillian returned to our porch from the Homecoming dance, Ryan offered a swift, gentlemanly goodnight hug. Kerry and I watched from our bedroom window. Much later, we would learn that Ryan began referring to Jillian as "the girl of my dreams" on that first date.

It was a nice thought, on an enchanted evening. At about midnight, Kerry and I kissed our suddenly bigger little girl goodnight.

"I love my life," Jillian said.

Kerry hung the teal dress in Jillian's closet. Not long ago, we fished it out from the pack of at least a dozen formal dresses our daughter has worn over the years. Long dresses for proms, short dresses for Homecomings. It still sparkled.

CHAPTER 16

Kelly

How old are those guys, Dad?
—KELLY

Meantime, Kelly was a senior in high school, and we worried about him. Typical teenaged-kid worries. *How are your grades? Where's your homework? Who do you think you're talking to? Look at me when I'm talking to you. Don't look at me that way. I'm not telling you again. Where are you going, what are you doing and who are you doing it with? When will you be back? When'd you get home last night? Where'd you put my car keys? No, I don't have twenty dollars. I'm your father, not your maid. Get out of the shower. Water costs money. You broke what? Don't tell me you forgot. Do you have to wear your hat that way? Those aren't shoes, my friend, unless you're Jesus. Get a haircut. As long as you live under my roof . . . I can't do it for you. How many times do I have to tell you? Pull your pants up.*

Turn the music down. Have you been drinking? Don't drink and drive. Be home by midnight.

Navigating adolescence is hazardous in any family. Trying it when your focus is on another child is even harder. Because this is a certifiable fact:

Sometime between about eighth grade and high school graduation, the connection is lost, and your child stops talking to you. He seeks refuge in everything he doesn't want you to know and hangs out with everyone who thinks just like he does. He doesn't understand that all you really want is a decent conversation.

I wrote about Kelly occasionally in the newspaper. I called him "The Kid Down the Hall." It seemed a properly vague reference to a typical teenager who sought nothing more than estrangement from his parents. Starting at age 14, he began digging a tunnel to his own personal China, deeper and deeper, marking each new excavation with a No Trespassing sign.

I can't tell you why the getting-along was easier with Jillian than with Kelly, but it was. Guys are guys. Guys don't share much of anything, really—especially when one is the father and the other is the teenaged son. The father-son dynamic is perpetual grist for fiction writers. Bookstores offer shelves of self-help, promising peaceful answers to the father-son wars. Those volumes are often larded with goopy sentiment: Fathers playing catch with sons. Or they are written by people with more postgraduate degrees than actual sons to raise.

When Kelly was 14 and 15 years old, I didn't have much of a connection with him beyond yelling at him. Dealing with Jillian was uncomplicated, partly because she was uncomplicated. Dealing with Kelly was like working a Rubik's Cube. In an irony only a parent can understand, Kelly became a bigger project than Jillian.

I'd tried various ways to reconnect with my Kid Down the Hall. I got him into wrestling, a sport I'd practiced with mild success for several years. He wrestled. He didn't like it.

I'd try to engage him in sports talk. After all, that was my job, and I knew a little about it. He had no interest in sports talk. Or sports generally.

Kelly liked rap music. I thought "rap music" was an oxymoron. No father-son conversation there. I decided I'd introduce him to some real music. Rock and roll. I commanded my 14-year-old to sit as I slipped some Rolling Stones into the CD player. I played "Gimme Shelter," and proclaimed it the "Greatest rock and roll song ever made." Keith Richards's opening guitar licks, menacing and taut, slid seamlessly into Mick Jagger's urgent vocal, considerably aided and abetted by Merry Clayton's feral wailing.

"A masterpiece," I announced at the finish. I was feeling pretty smooth.

I hoped my son would hear "Gimme Shelter" and begin a love affair with good music. That is, my music. Or at least I hoped he'd take a break from his current heroes, Tupac and Snoop Dogg. I thought an intro to the music I enjoyed at his age would forge a re-bond between us, just as he began his wade into the teenaged swamp. I really believed that.

"What did you think of that?" I asked. "Pretty awesome, wasn't it?"

I actually used the word "awesome" at age 42. No wonder kids think parents are ridiculous. I was planning on breaking out some Allman Brothers, a little Eagles, maybe some Hendrix. You think you're cool, kid? Check this out. It's awesome.

That's when Kelly said, "How old are those guys, Dad?"

He was a smart kid who didn't like school. "I like high school when I'm not there" was how he explained it. He was a respectful kid who nevertheless did what he pleased as much as possible, not all of it respectful and much of it undetected.

He was a friendly kid who kept a small circle of friends. Kelly didn't do school things. No dances, no football games, no clubs. He wasn't antisocial; he was selectively social. As Kelly put it, "Dances sucked. Homecoming sucked. Going to high school football games was cool. In middle school."

He always wanted to get away. Denver was a fascination for a time. Then the West Coast. Kelly didn't want to stay in Loveland, or Ohio. He believed the kids who thought high school was great were the kids who never left Loveland. By the time he was a senior, it didn't much matter where he went, as long as he could get away from here.

The deeper he got into high school, the more his grades retreated. He lacked motivation. He experimented with what high school kids experiment with. We sent him briefly to a psychologist. He wouldn't talk to us, not even disrespectfully. We thought he needed to talk to someone. He thought that was ridiculous.

"Do you have anything you'd like to talk about?" the doctor would begin.

"No."

"Why do you think you're here?"

"My parents made me come."

"No issues or concerns?"

"No."

Sixty minutes of silence ensued. Fairly quickly, the doctor announced she couldn't "help" Kelly.

"That's because there was nothing to help," he said.

In truth, there wasn't. We didn't know that then. We just saw a bright kid who didn't care about school. We didn't want Kelly to flush his future. We didn't know how to fix him. We yelled a lot. Kelly never yelled back. He never said anything. We wished he would say something. Anything.

"Do you understand?"

"Yes."

"We can't do the work for you. You have to want to change your life."

"I know."

"What are you going to do about it?"

"I'll do better. I guess."

All he wanted was for the lecture to end.

My dad was a yeller. He yelled so frequently that I became expert at tuning him out. I could tell what words he was yelling by the inflections in his voice. The up-and-down cadence let me know what the sermon was about. I didn't need to hear the words to know exactly what they were.

As I yelled at Kelly, I knew he was doing the same thing.

He sat politely and offered the good answers. Then he'd go to the basement, shut the door, engage the thump-thump of Tupac and enter a different place.

Turn the music down.

During those times, the lingering fear was that Kerry and I had neglected our son in service to our daughter. We didn't think we had. But building the better Jillian could be a soul-sapping enterprise. Emotional energy wasn't boundless.

"Do we need to spend more time with him?" Kerry would ask.

"He doesn't want to spend more time with us," I'd say.

"Then, what?" she'd ask.

I didn't know.

We believed that, in all the fundamental ways, we'd raised Jillian the same way we'd raised Kelly. We hadn't given her preferential treatment. She had responsibilities. She had to be respectful to us and to others. Jillian had to make her bed and clean her room. She had to help with the dinner dishes. When she messed up, we punished her. We may have allowed for her disability, but we didn't cater to it.

Occasionally, usually at the dinner table, Jillian would boast about something nice she'd done for someone at school that day. "You're the good child," we'd say, a teasing shot across Kelly's apathetic bow. Jillian would borrow the phrase whenever she and Kelly quibbled. "I'm the good child, Kelly," she'd say.

We had made a point of spending as much time with Kelly as we did with Jillian. When he was younger, he appreciated it, but by high school, he probably wished we would let that go. Kerry in particular had made sure Kelly felt fully included. Mothers and sons have the same bond as fathers and daughters. Kerry was always closer to our son than I was.

Yet there was no denying that we needed different approaches to raising each child. As Nancy Croskey had said, one size didn't fit all.

Kelly provoked different worries than Jillian. We'd never worry about the 3:00 a.m. phone calls with Jillian. We wouldn't listen for her opening the garage door on a Saturday night. Jillian could be typically teenaged in her attitude. But she didn't party. We always knew where she was. We walked the midnight floor worrying about her future. Not her present.

We worried about Kelly's present.

They're two very different people. Jillian is social, engaging and engaged. Kelly is contemplative. He taught himself to play the guitar. Hours in the basement, experimenting with sounds. It was Kelly's kind of thing, a solo accomplishment set to music. He's the guy in the corner at the party, observing and nursing a beer. That's if he goes to the party, which he'll do only under protest. A good day for him is a walk in the woods with a very good friend or his girlfriend, smoking a cheap cigar and now that he's legal, taking a nip of Jack Daniel's, before finishing the day listening to music.

Kelly has always loved reading. When he was a freshman in high school, I gave him a book of Hemingway short stories. "Read 'Big Two-Hearted River.' That'll tell you all you need to know about Hemingway," I said. Surprisingly, he did. Kelly didn't become a Hemingway devotee right away; that took years. But it was the story that piqued his interest.

He wrote his master's thesis on Hemingway and Fitzgerald. Discussion of "Big Two-Hearted River" consumed several pages.

Jillian is an open book. Kelly is a Faulkner novel. He's careful who he lets in. You can know him. It takes time. I've been working on it for 28 years.

To some extent, you raise your kids the way your parents raised you. My dad was an engaged parent, if not exceptionally attentive. We used sports as our adhesive. We had season tickets to Washington Redskins games. We spent that lost and lonely winter on the Greyhound to and from Baltimore, going to Bullets basketball games. We played catch, though not routinely, and only when I asked.

I tried the catch stuff with Kelly. I was always the instigator. It was comical, this nearly 40-something guy with a ball glove on his hand, beseeching his 10-year-old to come out and play.

Jillian had no such issues with her brother. To her, everything Kelly did was cool. There were times when Kelly felt the only person who loved him unconditionally was his

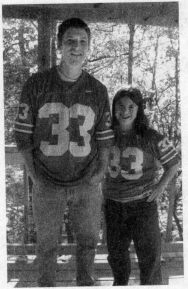

Kelly and Jillian at our cabin in rural Ohio.

little sister. She didn't care about the *D* he got on his report card. She knew he had parties when we were out of town. She knows things about her brother that Kerry and I will never know. They had a bond that Jillian's disability affected only in good ways. Kelly assumed the role of protector. He has said since that he would never have been as close to her if she were typical.

Kelly saw that we cut his sister no slack. He recognized

how she worshipped him and never doubted him. Love is love. Even for a teenager in full rebellion, it's hard to resist Jillian, especially if you know her more than a little. Kelly knew her a lot.

"I always loved Jillian," he said.

As for loving his parents . . . it was more from afar.

When he was 17 years old, Kelly moved his room into the basement. He spent most of his time down there. I'd get up at 3:00 a.m. for a drink of water, and the light would be on. Kelly stayed awake for days at a time, playing guitar and video games. At one point in high school, he wrote the word "LOST" on the wall of the basement.

"Why'd you do that?" I asked.

"It was part of a quote. From Chaucer."

"Chaucer?" My kid's quoting Chaucer?

"Introduction to the Man of Law's Tale," he said. "Lost money is not lost beyond recall. But loss of time brings on the loss of all."

Well, all right then.

"Do you feel lost?" I wondered, obliviously.

"No," Kelly said. "I'm broke."

But the thought gnawed at me: What to do with a lost son? With Jillian, it was easy: The Coffee Song, the walks to the bus, the immutable fact that I was Dad, and little girls love their dads. With Kelly, it was elusive, like eating soup with a fork.

Kerry came up with the answer. And like lots of answers involving your teenaged kid, there was a little desperation attached. We decided to spend our last dollar on a lottery ticket. What the hell.

We'd take a trip.

Kelly was 14 years old the first time I took him to Montreat, North Carolina. Montreat is a Presbyterian retreat about 15 miles east of Asheville. It's God's country. Literally. The Rev. Billy Graham has lived there for at least half a century.

By the time I was 40 years old, I'd been going to Montreat on and off for 35 years. I'm not especially religious. But certain places affect us all in certain ways. Montreat blessed me with a spiritual peace I'd never found anywhere else. I felt I belonged there. It's hard to articulate that feeling. You just know it when you're in it.

Montreat progresses in geologic time. It changes about as obviously as the needles on a hemlock. I needed its constancy. I first went there with my birth mother. Then I went there the summer after she died with my grandparents, her parents, to grieve. The protective shoulders of the mountains afforded a place for my sad head. I tried to make it back every summer.

I'd lost touch with Montreat for several years, though. We'd lived in Dallas and New York, too far by car. When we moved to Cincinnati in 1988, the partnership resumed. Montreat was 400 miles by interstate. I started taking a few days there alone, to wander and ponder. Kelly came by his introspection genetically.

Kerry suggested I take him along. I hesitated.

"That's my time," I said. Still selfish, after all those years.

"Make time for your son."

The first few years, we didn't speak much. Neither of us enjoys lots of conversation anyway. The teen years were starting to take full effect. He really didn't have a lot he wanted to communicate with me. It was a six-hour drive, and we spent three nights in a bed and breakfast. We might have said 30 words.

We did what I liked because I wasn't worried about what he liked. We hiked Lookout Mountain in Montreat. We followed the ancient spine of the Blue Ridge Mountains to Craggy Gardens, where we carved our initials into the beam of a shelter, originally built by the Civilian Conservation Corps in 1934. We hiked down to the 100-foot sheer plume of Crabtree Falls. We visited Graveyard Fields, a mile-high meadow named for the stumps of trees felled by hurricane winds early in the last century. The tree stumps resembled headstones.

I told Kelly to watch out for bears, and that the blueberries along the trail were suitable for eating.

None of it seemed to interest him.

After two summers, I decided I'd had enough. It was awkward, I wasn't enjoying it. Kelly didn't seem to be either.

"I think I'm going alone next year," I told Kerry upon our return.

"Why?"

"Because we don't talk, and I'm tired of wondering if he has a good time."

"He loves going with you," Kerry said.

"What?"

"He has told me the last two years what a great time he has had."

I was stunned. I'd never heard a word. By the end of year two's trip, I'd assumed Kelly was going along to humor me. I had no idea.

That was Kelly. Rather, Kelly and me. Why do fathers and sons sometimes have such a hard time communicating? I could talk to Jillian all day. Kelly and I communicated in grunts.

"He has never said a thing to me about it," I told Kerry.

"Why don't you ask him?" she said.

Okay.

"Do you like going to Montreat?"

Yeah, Kelly said. He did.

"Really?"

"Yeah."

"Why don't you say anything?"

"I dunno."

"You want to go back next year?"

"Yeah."

"Do you think we might actually, you know, talk?"

Haha. "Maybe," Kelly said.

We kept going back. It got a little better each year. *He* got a little better each year. I'd lucked into a common love. I'd found a kindred spirit. I wasn't about to let it go. I'd find my kid again, one hike at a time.

We'd do the same things every visit. As we crossed the state lines from Tennessee to North Carolina on Interstate 40, I'd play the Van Morrison tune "Alan Watts' Blues." Morrison's mystical, wandering side comes through in this tune when he sings of finding solitude atop a mountain. "Cloud hidden," he calls it.

We'd head into Asheville at night to eat and wander the downtown streets. Over the past decade, Asheville has reinvented itself as a cultural mecca for young and creative people. Kelly enjoyed the hippie-esque vibe.

He'd still go silent occasionally. He'd leave the room at 11:00 p.m., to talk to his girlfriend for an hour on the phone. He'd also spend an hour talking with me. He even started listening to the Rolling Stones.

"Best Stones album," Kelly offered a few Augusts ago as we meandered down some half-forgotten North Carolina trail, 5,000 feet above the everyday. He had to be 24 years old by then. He was going to be a senior at Ohio State. He was majoring in English, making good grades. He'd met a girl and fallen in love.

"*Exile*," I said. *Exile On Main Street* was recorded in 1972, at a chateau in the south of France, where the Stones had fled to escape the high taxes of merry old England.

Kelly agreed, though he suggested *Beggars Banquet* was a close second.

"Not even in the photo," I said. "*Exile, Let It Bleed. Get Yer Ya-Ya's Out. Sticky Fingers.* Then, maybe *Beggars*."

I stopped for a second then, to ponder the wonder and irony of that conversation. A decade earlier, I'd played "Gimme Shelter" to Kelly's indifference. Now, we were debating Stones' albums as if we were critics.

We'd made a connection.

The cure for our ills was time and patience. Kelly and I will never be peers. But we have become friends. The tug-of-wills that defined our relationship when he was younger has abated. I enjoy him. I believe he feels likewise.

I have no idea if Kelly's rough seasons came in part from the necessary attention we paid his sister. He has said no. He was just being a teenaged boy. It doesn't much matter now. Now, we can see Jillian's good effect on him. And, maybe, our effect, too.

Kelly and I have been to Montreat every summer for the past 14 years, half of Kelly's life, willingly, as Van Morrison would put it, cloud-hidden. He emerged from the dismal swamp of high school, hardly worse for wear. He frayed Kerry and me some, but that was part of the parental deal. Kelly grew to be the person we'd hoped. I'd like to think that Montreat helped, that somewhere among those magical peaks, whereabouts unknown, my son and I found the adhesive of our lives, and it made a difference.

I will go to Montreat with him as long as I am able, and whenever he is available. I rue the summer when life decides we've had enough. Kelly sees Montreat now as I always have. It is my best gift to him.

My hope is that when I'm done, Montreat will remain an heirloom. Kelly will take his son there. Maybe their relationship will be cantankerous for a while. Maybe Kelly will see his son's silence as disapproval, when all it is is a coming of age.

Maybe he'll think of abandoning the project. A wiser head will discourage that. He'll keep going, with his son, up the trail leading to the heath bald of Craggy Gardens, half in the clouds. They'll go to that place where in June, the Catawba rhododendrons bloom in bursts of red, like a five-alarm fire.

"This is where Grandpa and I used to come," he'll say. Maybe he'll point to the pair of initials cut into that great beam of wood in the shelter. *KD. PD.*

Kelly will nod then and catch the lump in his throat. He'll know how I felt, all those years ago. Just wanting a conversation.

Kelly and I groped for a long time because groping is often what fathers and sons do. That would have been true, regardless.

Ultimately, with time, patience and time spent cloud-hidden, Kelly became the man we knew he could be.

CHAPTER 17

An Appropriate Education

*Any parent who has a child that's different
has a right to be irrational.*
—BUZZ BISSINGER

Jillian arrived at Loveland High School an excited and enthusiastic freshman. As she had with previous milestones, Jillian
reminded me that she wasn't my little girl anymore. "Your little
girl is growing up," she'd say.

"You could be Father Time and you'd still be my little girl,"
said I.

School buildings changed, but Jillian's academic issues did
not. Her biggest struggle was reading. Jillian struggled in ninth
grade with the same words she tripped over in sixth grade.
That indicated two possibilities:

Jillian had maxed out her reading potential.

Her teachers weren't doing all they could.

Teachers said Jillian worked hard. The summaries of her test results always came with qualifiers. Jillian is "actively involved." Her "focus and attention" rarely stray. She "wants to do well and seems always to do her best." However, Jillian "struggles with the main idea and struggles with concrete and abstract questions." Jillian "struggles with summaries." In general, Jillian works hard but struggles to comprehend anything. She reads words. She doesn't know what they mean.

Kerry and I were not convinced Jillian could become a better reader, but we were determined to do everything we could to give her a chance. What we wanted cost thousands of dollars a year for private, individual instruction. The law clearly says that if a school cannot provide an in-house service that a student requires, the school is obligated to pay for that service elsewhere.

When Jillian was a freshman, Ellen Mavriplis suggested we enroll her in a specialized program at a local reading center, where Jillian would get one-on-one training for two hours a day. The high school simply couldn't provide that.

The Langsford Learning Acceleration Center claimed to have "proven results teaching phonemic awareness, phonics, reading, spelling and comprehension, using specialized, research-proven approaches." Ellen convinced us of the effectiveness of Langsford. Ryan had already been going there for two years.

We said okay. Then we looked at the cost and flinched. The going rate at the Langsford Center was $65 an hour: Ten hours a week, for roughly 30 weeks. Thirty weeks, at $650 a week. Even a sportswriter knew that math: $19,500 a school year, not including the summer session.

Our gulps must have been audible. "You're entitled to this," Ellen said.

We might have been. The school system was not going to rubber-stamp it. The district superintendent at the time, Kevin Boys, claimed that each special-needs student cost a school district three times more to educate than a typical student. Meantime, Boys said, the federal government was bearing only 28 percent of the cost.

That gave Kerry and me pause, even as we fought for the money. Boys's job was to spend tax money efficiently. Spending thousands of extra dollars on one student was inefficient. No matter what the law said.

There were times when I agreed with Boys. I thought we were selfish. What makes our child so special? I believed we were somewhat hypocritical. We wanted Jillian entirely included in regular classrooms and treated the same as her peers. And yet, we demanded that her disability be given special dispensation because that was the law.

Who were we to have it both ways?

I was ambivalent as we went to the IEP meetings and asked for more. By the time Jillian entered high school, Ellen had become our advocate and participated fully in the meetings. Blunt, candid and wise to the fine points of the law, Ellen was a formidable presence on our side of the table.

We even brought Jillian to a meeting. We wanted her to experience fighting for herself. We wanted her to articulate what she wanted from her high school experience. We coached her a little the night before the meeting.

"You need to tell them you are your own advocate," Kerry said. "You want to graduate from high school and go to college.

You want to be a preschool teacher and get married to your boyfriend and have your own apartment."

At the meeting, Jillian was pitch-perfect. "I am my own a'vocate," she said. "I love high school, but I'm growing up. I'm not my dad's little girl anymore. I'm looking forward to college, and the rest of my life. I want my own 'partment."

When Jillian finished, the special-education director resumed debating the reading program. It was as if Jillian hadn't been there. We thought Jillian's presence might have had an impact. It didn't.

The district agreed to adopt the reading program Jillian's freshman year, with the condition it be taught at school, by someone already employed by the district. They'd pay to send a teacher to a conference to learn the program. They would not pay for the Langsford Center. We compromised and hoped for the best.

That year was not successful. The special-education teacher charged with helping Jillian had minimal training. Her workload didn't allow for the two hours daily that was required. At the outset of Jillian's sophomore year, we asked again that she attend the Langsford Center.

The district people agreed, but only after we filed a due process claim against the district that it would almost certainly lose. Jillian went to Langsford her sophomore year. Her junior year, we fought to have her continue there. And so on.

As a gesture of goodwill, Kerry and I even agreed that when we felt Jillian's progress had leveled off, we would recommend that she no longer needed to attend Langsford. School officials took issue with the progress Jillian had made while enrolled at Langsford. Everyone came to the IEPs Jillian's junior year

armed with statistics. Ellen brought test results from Langsford. All these percentiles, represented by clean, easy-to-read
bar graphs, accompanied by technical headings. *Manipulat-
ing Syllables. Auditory Conceptualization Test.* Big words for
simple tasks.

"I just don't see it," the district's special-ed director said.

"It's right there," Ellen said. On that bar graph. Et cetera.
As the parent at this juncture, you feel like leaving your skin.
I should have brought the Meyerowitz photograph to wish
myself into.

The district had its own numbers. They indicated that Jillian was not benefiting from the extra work.

Jillian's "intervention specialist" at school has written an
"IEP Progress Report." In one neatly arranged column, it lists
"Goal/Objective." In the next are the dates during which Jillian
strived to meet that Goal/Objective, and how she did. Here is
one of six Goal/Objectives in the progress report:

> Jillian will develop independent reading skills with in-
> creased vocabulary, word recognition, fluency, and uti-
> lize effective strategies for comprehension.

Here's the comment regarding her advancement:

> Making adequate progress.

Oh. Compared to what? All six of Jillian's Goal/Objectives
included that phrase.

Utilize effective strategies for comprehension. What does that
mean? What are the strategies? How do we know they're effective?

Jillian seems to enjoy writing was another assessment. Well, great. Is she making adequate progress in her enjoyment? If so, well, so what?

The Langsford conclusions were more detailed. They sounded more considered. They were also self-serving: *"We recommend that Jillian continue to receive one-to-one, intensive sessions . . ."*

That's because, as the Langsford people suggest, *"One-to-one sessions are important because these programs are retraining Jillian's brain. Jillian needs the freedom to work at her own pace. Group instruction would not allow this flexibility."*

And finally: *"We recommend Jillian receive a minimum of 200 to 240 hours of sessions before evaluating her again to determine progress and make [a] decision about her next phase of treatment."*

Two hundred and forty hours? What is Jillian's "next phase"? Reading *Ulysses* over a long weekend?

It was during times such as this, an hour deep into the IEP morass, that I allowed myself to wonder: What if the school district people are right? What if the school people are the ones making sense here? Are we pushing it?

Maybe Jillian has maxed out. She is a junior. She has been attending sessions at Langsford for more than two years. The Langsford bar graphs show decided improvement. The school's numbers say just the opposite. We read with Jillian at home, and we're not sure what to think. Is she comprehending more and better? She's reading more words correctly. Does she understand their meanings? Is she establishing a base that will allow her to grasp the nuances and distinctions inherent in anything she reads that doesn't feature pictures?

By extension: Should we stop pushing so forcefully for further classroom education? Maybe Jillian's future should not include college. A vocational program might be more fitting. We want to prepare her for a life of independence. Should that include higher education or job training?

My old familiar doubts came calling: Whose dream is it?

This is what I wonder as Ellen and Kerry face off with the school people. Then I think of Jillian. How hard she works. "One more time," she'll say as we slog through history questions at 10:00 p.m. on a school night. Why not give Jillian the opportunity she has earned?

I'm not going to limit her. Why should I allow anyone else to?

"Can I say something?" I ask.

"Go right ahead," the special-ed director says.

My passion is always new, even as my words are rote. I go on for several minutes: Look at Jillian, don't see her . . . she wants to learn . . . she wants to please you . . . an opportunity, not a burden . . . she'll help you as much as you help her. I close with, "Those of you who look at Jillian as someone with Down syndrome aren't seeing the child who can help make you a better teacher and person, while you give her the education to which she's legally entitled."

"Can we all turn to page seven of the IEP?" the special-ed director asks.

"You might even be glad when Jillian leaves here," I continue. "But we're not the last family you're going to have to deal with in the coming years. We're the first. So you might as well figure out something that works for everyone."

"Thank you, Mr. Daugherty," the special-ed guy says. His

face betrays no emotion. He asks if we could all turn the page. He means the IEP summary.

The law forced the school district to pay for services it might not have had the money for. "I'm a teacher," Kerry said then. "I understood there are only so many minutes in a day, and that school districts only have so much money."

If the fight were just about money, we'd have closed our mouths and opened our wallets. We could afford the $40,000, or whatever the cost ended up being. At its core, the struggle was about perception.

Kevin Boys cast an accountant's eye at the proceedings. Boys felt compassion for Jillian. But not so much that he wouldn't fight us to save money. As he admitted a few years after Jillian graduated from high school, "It boils down to money and how you spend it. Nobody's going to tell you that. Not having money is not an acceptable reason not to do something.

"When that law was originally passed in the '70s, there was an expectation it would be funded at a certain level. That hasn't happened. What happens is, the local school district picks up the rest. That's a financial challenge. As a school superintendent, I champion offering optimal programs for our kids. But that's not my job. My job is to provide a good education for our kids, given the resources we have.

"The special education law doesn't say we're supposed to provide an optimal education. It says we're supposed to provide a free and appropriate education. If I want to provide optimal education for my son, it'd look a lot different and cost a lot more.

"There's the expectation you provide the optimal education. You don't have the resources."

"You're saying we were unrealistic in what we expected for Jillian," I said to Boys.

"A lot of parents are unrealistic," Boys said.

This is what happens when a family's dreams collide head-on with a school system's priorities.

During Jillian's junior year, Kevin Boys made an entirely unexpected appearance in the gym, where Kerry was teaching a class. We'd threatened due process, yet again.

Boys handed her an envelope. "I'd rather do this than pay for lawyers," he said. The envelope contained a signed memorandum, stating that the district would pay for Jillian's time at Langsford for the rest of that year.

We were happy, but not elated. Happy that Jillian would at least get the chance to be a better reader. Less than elated that we'd spent so long working at cross-purposes, at Jillian's expense. I still wonder if my competitiveness served my daughter or hindered her. I wanted the reading program. I also wanted to win.

Times change. Hopefully, we progress. What worked 30 years ago doesn't work now. Some of Jillian's biggest wins came at school. Also, some of our most enduring sadness. It depended on who was looking, and who was seeing.

Meantime, the seemingly endless struggle produced repercussions beyond the IEP conference room. In the spring of Jillian's junior year, the principal tried to fire my wife.

Not fire, exactly. Kerry was offered a new one-year contract. In the 11 years she'd been teaching Health and Physical Education at the high school, Kerry always had worked with three-year deals. This was standard for any established teacher. The one-year offer was a shot across Kerry's bow.

The message was clear: You have caused trouble around here. Here's your new contract. Enjoy. It was clumsy and vengeful, and we had been expecting it. In our effort to get Jillian an education, Kerry and I became a general nuisance to those who ran the school district. They didn't like us. They wanted us to go away. That's how Kerry had ended up in the principal's office, summoned like a sophomore who'd set a bathroom trash can on fire.

"Come up and see me at the end of the day," the principal said.

Kerry went. "We're reducing you to a one-year contract," the principal told her.

Kerry asked why. The principal cited an instance in which Kerry hadn't supervised the locker room carefully enough and, because of that, money was taken from a student's gym locker. She said that students "didn't seem happy" coming to Kerry's Phys Ed class. She said Kerry "didn't socialize enough" with the other teachers.

Well, okay. Kerry responded that she had been teaching a class when the money was stolen, and she couldn't be watching the locker room at the same time. She didn't understand what the principal meant by unhappy kids. She said it was hard to socialize with teachers she'd criticized during IEP meetings. It was uncomfortable for everyone.

And really, since when is not socializing a reason to have a contract shortened?

"This is about Jillian, isn't it?" Kerry asked the principal.

"That's just the attitude I'm talking about," the principal said.

Apparently, fighting for your child's education is having an "attitude."

The principal denied it had anything to do with Jillian. That was laughable.

Kerry contacted her union representative the same day the principal offered the one-year contract, and shortly thereafter, she and the rep met with the principal, armed with ten years of excellent teacher evaluations. Nothing changed. The rep filed a grievance on Kerry's behalf, against the principal, and another against the district. Kevin Boys backed his principal. A mediator was summoned. Our fight with Loveland Schools rolled on, in a different direction. It wasn't just the aides and teachers who occasionally looked at Jillian and saw problems and not opportunities.

The previous October, Kerry and I had met with the principal in her office, in yet another attempt at locating the elusive, happy middle between learning and learning under budget. It didn't work, of course. The school was in business to save money, not to spend it on Jillian. Due process comes into play when parents sue the school district for not following the law, as it applies to providing an education to a student with a disability. The cases can be long and costly. Ellen Mavriplis, Ryan's mother and founder of Inclusion Advocates, says schools win these cases more often than not.

That said, districts often prefer to settle if the cases against them are solid, as was the case with Jillian.

Money was an issue, but mainly as a symbol: The school district felt Jillian wasn't worth the expense. Jillian was an inconvenience. Now Kerry was, too. It was during those times that frustration assumed in me a living presence. It became as much a part of me as my hands and feet.

"You've failed my daughter," I told the principal on that

October day. I looked her dead in the eye, with all the polite malice I could muster. Diplomacy isn't my best trait, and after years of IEP meetings, I wasn't in a congenial mood. So I said it again, in case she'd missed it the first time.

You've failed my daughter.

If that hit the principal the same way "Jillian can't learn"— uttered by a speech therapist at an IEP meeting Jillian's junior year—had hit me, well, there you go.

Later, after I'd left the building, the principal looked at Kerry from across her desk. "Tell him not to say that," she said. A school levy loomed on the November ballot. Election Day was less than a month away.

Everyone at Loveland High School knew I worked at the *Cincinnati Enquirer*. But the school people didn't know me well enough to know I'd never use my position to further a personal cause. I had opinions, but I didn't offer them from the bully pulpit. I would never editorialize publicly on their shortcomings, but I would tell someone who might. The levy was critical. No one connected with the schools wanted bad publicity.

"I'm not telling him anything," Kerry replied.

Saying what I did that day didn't come easily. Jillian attended school there. It was where Kerry drew a paycheck. But even more difficult was understanding why I needed to say anything at all. This was 2007. IDEA was 32 years old. Middle-aged. It should have evolved from an ideal to a policy to a respected truth.

It's hard being Daniel Boone. We heard often from other parents of children with disabilities who hadn't stomped their feet. They were grateful and slightly amazed. Compared to earlier generations of parents of kids with disabilities, Kerry and I were moving heaven and earth. And compared with earlier years, Loveland High was doing some of the same, even though it wasn't enough. Parents praised our trail blazing. We appreciated their support. Sometimes, we just wanted to take off our backpacks and boots and rub the soreness.

Kerry and her union representative would meet again with the principal and other school officials regarding her stunted contract. Soon enough, the school people saw they didn't have a case because Kerry's record had been exemplary. The charges were heavy-handed coercion.

Kerry agreed to a one-year deal, with a two-year extension.

The principal received a formal reprimand from the school district, and Kerry's case was brought up during the next labor negotiation between teachers and the district. The result was a ruling that a school principal could no longer reduce the length of a teacher's contract without proper documentation.

The union rep asked Kerry if she'd like a written apology from the principal, but she declined. It wasn't necessary. Everyone knew who was right. And who wasn't.

All because of a disagreement over how an eager student should be educated. By the middle of Jillian's senior year, Kerry and I decided Jillian's reading progress had leveled off. We informed the school that we'd no longer need the extra services at the Langsford Center. We thanked everyone for what they'd done.

CHAPTER 18

Belonging

She genuinely cares about other people.
—EVAN STANLEY

The irony was, Jillian was doing beautifully. She had no idea her trailblazing parents were rubbing their feet. Jillian would not have understood anyway. She had neither the heart nor the intellect to question people's best intentions. The thought that her teachers would be anything less than entirely enthusiastic on her behalf wouldn't register with her.

One day after school in her sophomore year, Jillian announced she had to be back at school at 5:00 p.m.

"What for?" Kerry asked.

"I have my dance team tryouts."

This was the first we'd heard about this. Jillian had seen the sign-up sheet and added her name. She'd never been on a team. She'd never danced publicly. Most of Jillian's dancing was done in her room, during the Jillian Daugherty Show.

She auditioned for the junior varsity team. The girls entertained during half-time at the JV basketball games. They wore skimpy outfits that made their grandparents blush. They danced to rock and hip-hop that was played over a scratchy PA system, minded by students who sometimes forgot to start the music on time, or at all.

Kerry recruited a varsity dancer to perform the JV routine, which Kerry videotaped. She gave the video to Jillian. We moved a full-length mirror into the basement. Jillian reprised the JD Show, this time to music. She spent hours practicing. Her two-wheeler mind-set was at work again, this time indoors. Early in the tryouts, the JV coach had suggested to Kerry that Jillian could be on the team—as the student charged with cuing the music. Kerry politely said that Jillian was either good enough to dance or she wouldn't be on the team.

As it was, there were no cuts, so Jillian made the team. Was she good enough?

Mostly, yes. She was coordinated; she had rhythm. Had Jillian been a typical kid, she'd have been an athlete. It's true there were times during the dance team's routines when she was a fraction of a second behind. If you looked only at Jillian, you'd notice. No parents looked only at Jillian, except Jillian's parents. They were all busy looking at their own children.

It didn't matter to them if the execution was jittery. Their kids were great.

Jillian worked tirelessly at learning the routines. She would come home, grab a snack and head to the basement. "I do my dance practice now." She'd start the music and square up to the mirror. She'd dance.

If I had to hear Aerosmith and Run-DMC do "Walk This Way" one more time, I was going to personally kidnap Steven Tyler and make him listen to Pat Boone.

Hour after hour, thumping around the basement room. *Just gimme a kiss . . .*

Jillian wasn't as good as the best dancers, and she never would have made the varsity team. But she was fearless, and she wasn't at all self-conscious. She danced for joy.

We would not have allowed Jillian to dance if we didn't know she could keep up. It wouldn't have been fair to her or to her teammates. The last thing we wanted as parents was to put Jillian in a position where she embarrassed herself. The dance had to look good. If it didn't, and Jillian was the reason, she'd ruin it for everyone. The dance never looked bad.

Years later, in college, Jillian would say, "I really miss my dance team." She'd ask if she could try out for her college's team. We said no. We told her she wasn't good enough. Sometimes, even parents wanting more than anything to let their daughter define herself had to step in and do some of the defining.

Jillian's dance teammates treated her like the rest of her typical peers did: Arm's-length pleasant. They didn't mind having her on the team. But I don't think they relished it either. They included her in team functions; pre-game dinners, sign-painting, that sort of thing. After practice or games, they went their ways, and Jillian went home. We didn't know if the girls hung out together after practice. We never asked.

Jillian loved to dance though. She did it well enough to belong.

That was her way of participating in extracurriculars. Jillian's will and joy always overrode any thoughts of not being more fully included by her teammates.

Jillian also set Loveland High School records for weightlifting. The sight of this four-foot-eight, 100-pound child deadlifting barbells was amusing and bizarre. She loved lifting—and she especially loved being around lots of boys. She liked wearing sweats, T-shirts and a backward baseball cap. She also got a kick out of the plaque on the weight room wall that proved she held school records for squat, bench press and deadlift. Just because there weren't a lot of 100-pound people lifting heavy weights didn't make Jillian think her records were anything less than awesome.

She liked athletes and referred to her favorites as her "homeys." Bobby Capobianco, a six-foot-seven center who would go on to play college ball at Indiana, and then Valparaiso, was a homey. Brian Wozniak, a football player at Loveland and then at the University of Wisconsin, was a homey. And then there was Evan Stanley.

Evan wasn't just a homey. In Jillian's orbit, he was her "home dog," a name so special she reserved it only for him. Before school started in the mornings, Jillian would wait for her home dog at the back entrance to the school, the entrance that was closest to the student parking lot. That's where they'd meet and walk to class.

I asked Jillian once what they talked about, and she said, "Our lives."

As the parent of a child with Down syndrome, I've heard lots of people tell me things like, "She's happy all the time." "She enjoys every day." "She's positive." "She makes me laugh." I've heard these descriptions so often they can come off as patronizing, depending on who's doing the praising. It can often sound saccharine and thin. *What a nice little girl she is*. It makes Jillian sound like a golden retriever.

Evan said a lot of those things too, but he wasn't patronizing her. He had known Jillian since they were in grade school together. Jillian had made sure they were more than just acquaintances by the time they were seniors at Loveland High. Jillian had lots of acquaintances. Just about every kid in school, basically. But Evan was really her friend, and she was his. He got something from the transaction. His other friends were quick to talk about themselves; Jillian wanted to talk about Evan: *What's new? How are things at basketball practice? How are your mom and dad? How's your girlfriend?*

Evan saw their morning walk to class as the highlight of his day because Jillian was selfless, in a setting not known for it. "It's refreshing to have someone like that in your life. She genuinely cares about other people," Evan said.

To Evan, Jillian was J-Dog. To Jillian, Evan was her link to typical. She never mentioned her disability, let alone lamented it. But she knew its shackles. In the court of peer opinion, she didn't win a lot, but when she did, she soaked it in. She was never more alive than when she was with Evan and her homeys.

Some of Jillian's best high school memories involved her support of her guys. She'd ask for a hall pass to use the girl's room, but instead go to the attendance office, where home dog Evan and homey Bobby worked. At the Loveland home basketball games, she'd make us get there early so she could be sure she'd get a seat in the first row, behind the team bench, so she could scream encouragement while these guys played.

She made Kerry and me sit deep in the bleachers, far away and anonymous.

Bobby was the star. Brian played a lot. Evan was, as Jillian put it, "my benchwarmer guy." That didn't stop her from lobbying the coach to play him. "Coach, coach! Put in Evan! He's my dog!"

That's when Evan would turn from his well-worn spot on the bench and shoot his biggest fan a look that shouted, *"Jillian, you're going to get me in trouble."*

Jillian's penchant for hanging with athletes, and modeling their behavior and tastes in music and fashion, endured into her college years. Her idea of dressing up was tucking in her Loveland Tigers Basketball T-shirt. "Pull your shorts up" was as routine a high school directive from Kerry and me as "clean your room."

From her homeys, Jillian developed a sense of belonging. Also an unfortunate taste for hip-hop and rap. Just because Jillian owned an intellectual disability didn't curb her enthusiasm for Eminem and Snoop Dogg. Kerry and I had Bobby and Evan to thank for that slice of atonal hell emanating from the basement of the house.

"Yo, Pops," Jillian might offer, when addressing me.

"I beg your pardon?"

"Oh, sorry," she'd say. "I mean, hey, Dad."

High school was a happy time for Jillian, in no small part because of her typical friends. One of them would cap Jillian's whole high school experience with one defining gesture just as all of them were preparing to leave.

CHAPTER 19

Jillian and Ryan

I promise to be good to your daughter, sir.
—RYAN

I love that boy.
—JILLIAN

I'd been replaced. That was plain. Forget the daily treks to the school bus stop, the Coffee Song, the reminders that Jillian was no longer my "little girl." That was nothing. I'd become Number Two on what Jillian called her Best Boy List. As in, "Ryan's my best boy now, Dad."

That first Homecoming date had become much more. Weekends were scheduled around their dates. Most kids with Down syndrome don't drive, nor do their friends with Down syndrome. If they're going to go anywhere together, someone has to take them. Kerry and I and Ellen and Dimitri were the designated drivers. After a few months, we decided we'd better paint our cars yellow and install meters on the dashboards.

This was not going to be a two-person relationship; it would require a six-person team. All of Jillian's life had been a collaboration. This new chapter would be no different. Jillian and Ryan were capable of having an abiding relationship, but they required a lot of help. They didn't necessarily want Kerry, Paul, Ellen and Dimitri around, but they most definitely needed us.

If they went to dinner, we went to dinner. When they went to the Cincinnati Reds game we did, too. Friday night or Saturday night was date night. For kids and adults. The adults were grateful that the kids liked Chinese. It was a good thing we were of like minds when it came to Jillian and Ryan. Our goals were entirely in sync. It was a happy coincidence that our children fell madly for each other.

Kerry and I lost friends in the Down syndrome community because of the way we'd chosen to raise Jillian. Other friends simply drifted away. Dimitri and Ellen were different. Like Kerry, Ellen had seen a calling realized when her son was born with Down syndrome. Kerry wanted to be a mother; Ellen wanted to be an advocate. It just hadn't happened for either of them the way they had originally envisioned.

Ellen knew what she wanted for Ryan's education, and she came to know the law. She would not be bullied or patronized. The school people she faced across the conference table might have said she was the one who did the bullying. "I don't accept what others say, unless I think it's just," she said. Dimitri concurred: "The unfairness of others drives her."

Very early in Jillian and Ryan's relationship, they requested that during their dates they'd appreciate the adults sitting as far away from them as possible. In the kitchen, perhaps, or in a different country. For the first year or so, we went where they went, but eventually we would simply drop them off and entertain ourselves elsewhere.

"I am here to take your daughter to a lovely dinner, sir," Ryan would announce when he arrived.

I would pound a fist to a palm in mock menace. "You better be good to her, young man," I'd say, whap-whap-whap.

"Oh, sir. I love your daughter. I always take good care of her."

And he did. He'd open doors for her—to the car, to the restaurant, to the house. On special occasions, he'd arrive with a spray of flowers. Ryan didn't show up at our front door in ragged blue jeans slung so low on his hips you could see his boxers. He didn't look away when you spoke to him, or act as if you were old and ridiculous. He dressed nicely. He smiled. He shook hands. He made conversation.

Our relationship with Dimitri and Ellen grew apace. For a while, disability conversation dominated. It was therapeutic. It was also easy to see, early in our friendship, that Ellen Mavriplis was not to be underestimated. She'd always had a rebel streak and an affinity for the underdog. In high school, she protested against nuclear power. In college, she majored in psychology. Difference attracted her.

"I had a passion for those who were socially outcast. I never shied from non-traditional thinking," she said.

She wanted to find a cure for autism. She married Dimitri, who had come to the states from Greece as a 20-year-old, speaking English as a second language, to get a college education at Ohio University. Before Ryan was born, Ellen had considered adopting a child with Down syndrome.

Eventually, Ellen would start her own business, Inclusion Advocates, to help the parents of children navigate the special-education system in the public schools.

More than anything, Ellen is competitive. She wants to win. When she is right, she wants it known. She has an edge that works very well in a confrontational setting, such as an IEP meeting. For Ellen, "advocate" is as much a verb as a noun. She could never have known how her passion would be tested and validated. And then she had Ryan. Some people spend their entire adult lives seeking professional fulfillment. Ellen found hers the day Ryan was born.

That day, a social worker came to Ellen's hospital room and urged her "not to make any decisions right away." Translation: Giving Ryan up for adoption is an option. Ellen had an easy answer: "Thank you. Now go away." She and Dimitri had no denial when Ryan was born. They were angry, but only at the reactions of others. They received sympathy; they didn't want it. They didn't much understand it. They had a beautiful baby.

Again the thoughts of Ellen and Dimitri paralleled our own. In the days after Ryan was born, they wanted to see success stories. Ellen said, "Give us the possibilities. There is going to be success. How do I make that happen? Don't tell me what Ryan might not do. Why would I aspire to the low end?"

An aunt sent Ellen a newspaper story about a young woman with Down syndrome who was bilingual and played tennis. It stuck with Ellen because of the hope it portrayed. "What else can these kids do? If we don't put limits on them, what can they achieve?"

After the trauma of the first day—"All I want is for people to love him," she told a cousin on the phone—Ellen started gathering her wits and her will. The family moved to South Bend, Indiana, soon after Ryan was born. Ellen joined the local Down syndrome support group there. The rebel had found a cause.

She met with the school system's director of student services. That's not unusual for a parent to do, but Ryan was barely a toddler. She wanted full inclusion at a time when full inclusion was the law, but not always the convention. "That was the only option," she said.

She became president of the local Down syndrome support group. She changed its name and its mission to include advocacy. That involved challenging the educational system. She helped form a task force of teachers, administrators, parents and local business leaders. The mission was to get the schools in line with IDEA. "I pulled out the law," she said. "I started researching. My mission was to do everything we possibly could to enhance Ryan's life."

Her approach was blunt: "This is what the law says. Here's what my son is entitled to. I want full inclusion. What are we going to do about it?" She got the ball moving in South Bend, then the family returned to Cincinnati when Ryan was three years old.

By then, he was a rambunctious preschooler. Ellen and Dimitri would open one side of Ryan's crib to allow him to come and go. He'd climb out and proceed to take all his books from the shelf and pile them in his crib, where he'd sit quietly and flip the pages.

Ellen enrolled Ryan in a Montessori school. By law, the public schools still had to provide him with services: Occupational and speech therapies, a classroom aide. The Mavriplises switched him to public school in third grade. Between fourth and fifth grades, the school wanted to move Ryan to a special-ed classroom. Before that happened, Ellen asked to observe one.

"It made me physically sick," she recalled. "The lowered bar, the watered-down behavior and academic expectations. Adults treating students like babies. So much unrealized potential. The kids in that classroom had no books. This was fifth grade."

Ryan's IEP dictated that he would be in a regular-ed classroom. The school brass couldn't change that without a due process hearing. No one wanted that, least of all school brass. The law was not on their side. "Let's not waste time talking about things that aren't going to happen," Ellen said. "Let's talk about how we're going to make this work."

What followed was eight years of persistence, vigilance and the imposition of Ellen's will. In Ryan's IEP meetings, she was direct, polite, forceful and intimidating. It helped that she stood just under six feet tall and knew the details of IDEA like an ant knows a picnic. She competed. "I dove into it. It was all about inclusion for me. Nothing else made sense."

We've debated over the years with me playing devil's advocate. Sometimes, I've actually believed what I've said.

"The feds have given this mandate to the states to give our kids a free and appropriate education," I might say. "But they haven't suggested how the states pay for it. I want Jillian educated. I'm willing to use the law as a sledgehammer. I'm also realistic. What if they don't have the money? What if the school district is tapped out?"

Ellen didn't care. She was not one for reasons, most of

which she saw as excuses. "They can spend it now, or they can spend it later," she would say. "If we skimp up front on their education, we pay far more to take care of them the rest of their lives."

It was cheaper to educate kids with disabilities than it was not to. Educate them, and they have a fighting chance to become productive, tax-paying members of society. Warehouse them in segregated classrooms, sheltered workshops and group homes, and they're likely to be on the government dole as long as they live.

"There aren't special lines at the grocery store," Ellen said. "Just because Ryan and Jillian have a disability doesn't mean they're less. They're different. We're all different."

"What if the schools don't have the money?" I persisted.

"Our society has made a commitment to take care of our citizens with disabilities," Ellen would say.

Three times, she and Dimitri filed due process cases on Ryan's behalf against stubborn school districts. Once, the district settled before the hearing. The other two times, Ellen won the case, and Ryan got the requested services.

Ellen turned the emotion she had for Ryan's situation into pure resolve. Emotion is just a start, she said. "Resolve gets results."

Kerry and I enlisted Ellen's services when Jillian was a sophomore in high school. Her knowledge of the law and her understanding of the IEP process added force to our argument with the school district. Ellen's presence at IEP meetings became mandatory and so meaningful that most meetings would end with school administrators asking if we intended to bring Ellen to the next meeting.

When we said yes, we knew the school folks would be bringing a lawyer or two.

We do our best work when we are inspired beyond ourselves. Ellen lived her work—and saw its results—every time Ryan walked through the door.

And now, he and Jillian would be walking hand-in-hand, to a restaurant or a movie or a ballgame. It appeared effortless. No agendas, jealousy or guile. No motives beyond enjoying this date and planning the next one. It has never been any different.

As Ellen put it, "He loves her. He really loves her." Because love is an emotion, it can be hard to articulate. Ellen gave it a good try.

"How do I describe that? They act like they're madly in love, every time they have a date. They have that essential quality that the rest of us spend our entire lives aspiring to. They love and accept each other unconditionally. With that comes respect. It's not an accident."

Long before Jillian met Ryan, she led with her heart. "I love my (fill in the blank)." Mom, Dad, Kelly. School, best friend Katie, Jake the guinea pig. Walker the dog. Her soccer team, her swim team, her neighborhood, her macaroni and cheese. Her life. Jillian expressed unconditional love for her life.

She wrote us notes. Hundreds, over the years. Sometimes they appeared after she'd done something wrong. For instance, after she'd spent her lunch money on candy and potato chips, Jillian wrote, "I so sorry about my lunch money. I love you guys. You are my heart and dreams."

Other times, she just wanted to express herself.

Dear Paul Daugherty:
  Thank you for be a great dad to me. I did have
fun with you all the time. It is so fun to be around
with you and take me to dinner with you. Oh last
thing, you are my heart and dreams and my best
father.

  Love, Jillian.

She'd slip the notes under the door of my office at home. They were handwritten at first. Then, as Jillian became accomplished on the computer, she'd type them and print them out. As she grew older, she switched to journals. A corner of her bedroom was filled with a stack of them, ten at least. Almost all the entries included the phrase "heart and dreams." Nothing Jillian wrote could leave her head without her heart's permission. Life, distilled and simplified. Heart and dreams: Don't leave home without 'em.

Four years to the day after they attended that first Homecoming dance, Jillian made dinner for Ryan. She was 18. He was 20. She set the table with a linen cloth and a bunch of freshly cut flowers. She lit candles. She inserted two pictures of her and Ryan into a snow globe.

Jillian wore a black dress, hem just above the knee. Her hair was pulled back and tied. She wore red lipstick, not too much. Makeup like stardust enhanced her gaze. She had bought the spaghetti and the meatballs and the cucumber for the salad. At close to 6:00, she stirred the sauce and tossed the salad. Ryan would arrive momentarily.

"I'm so excited," she said.

Ryan arrived, immaculate and announcing his good intentions. I whap-whap-whapped my fist to my palm, for what by then was easily the 500th time. "I love your daughter, sir," he said, also for the 500th time. He brought flowers and a bracelet bearing both of their names.

Kerry and I retreated upstairs to the foreign country of our bedroom, balancing our plates on our knees. We snooped a little.

Jillian and Ryan laughed at each other's jokes. "You're my best boy," Jillian said.

Ryan said, "Thank you. I'm afraid of your dad."

"Don't worry about it, Ryan," Jillian says.

"No. I am," Ryan says. From the top of the stairs we hear Ryan's fist slapping his palm. Whap-whap-whap.

"He just teasing you. But you love me, right?"

"Of course," Ryan says. Then he calls Jillian "darling."

Jillian yelled up the stairs when they were done: "You guys can come down now!" After dinner, Kerry cleans up. Jillian and Ryan slow dance to a country song.

Later, when Ryan has gone home and the night is bright with stars, Jillian and I sit on the deck out back, listening to the music of the night.

"Good time, sweets?" I ask.

"Yeah," she says. "You know what, Dad?"

"What?"

"I love that boy."

A few years later, on Valentine's Day, Jillian again makes dinner: Stuffed shells, salad, bread sticks. Kerry and I bring a folding table into the family room, in front of a fire we'd made for the occasion. Kenny G is on the CD player.

Ryan appears in a coat and tie, again bearing flowers. Jillian is in a brown dress, worn originally at a formal dance, a prom or a Homecoming in the not-too-distant past. Her closet is filled with formal dresses. It looks like a rainbow of finery.

They offer toasts.

Ryan, first: "I just want to say I love your daughter, and I am so happy I am with her tonight, having this wonderful dinner."

Then Jillian: "I so happy to be here with you guys and my best boy on Valentine's Day."

Sparkling grape juice all around, before the parents again retreat to the country upstairs, plates on laps.

Jillian and Ryan sit close on the coach, feet propped on the ottoman, watching the Disney Channel. They know how they feel. They know how they make each other feel. Their love is easy.

After a while, Jillian gives Kerry and me permission to come downstairs. She asks that I find "Goodnight, My Love" and put it in the CD player. After I pretend to be seriously aggrieved—"That's *our* song, Jills!"—I slip it into the machine. Jillian says thanks and tells me I can leave now.

Well, okay.

Later, after Jillian and Ryan say their goodbyes, Jillian asks me to put the song back on. She grabs my hand and pulls me onto the dance floor. Her head rests on my chest. "This never gets old," Jillian says. We dance to "Goodnight, My Love" in slow circles, all the way back to 1989.

Mister Number Two still draws the occasional glance from his Best Girl. She has moved on, and that is the way it should be. Number Two still gets that occasional wink, though.

JILLIAN AND RYAN LIVE their once-upon-a-times. They are who the street-corner poets wrote about in the still of the night. Their relationship informs us. We look at them and say, "This is how it can be."

A few days later, Jillian writes this:

> *Dear Ryan:*
> *I love you so much in my heart and this is*
> *amazing we are dating about 6 years. I have been*
> *thinking about our love and kisses too. We are*
> *wonderful together. I will make a love song for you.*

Ryan reads it, and reddens. "I love your daughter, sir," he says.

As the years have passed, we've loosened the leash. They've celebrated an anniversary with a dinner cruise on a stern-wheeler, where they delighted the other passengers with their dancing and, later, romancing on the deck of the boat as it plied the Ohio River past the city lights of Cincinnati.

We like to think the way we interpret their relationship is also glimpsed and appreciated by the rest of the world. Acceptance and respect aren't solely the province of "typical" couples. They can happen to anyone whose mind is open and whose heart is as willing as it is pure.

The Dells once sang, hopefully, that "Love is so simple." Most of us have disproved that pronouncement, through word and deed. We have regret and sadness. Not all of us, though. Not all of us.

Two years ago, Jillian and Ryan went to dinner at the Cheesecake Factory at a local shopping mall. Ryan appeared especially nervous as we drove them to the restaurant. "You okay, Ryan?" Jillian asked him. "Yeah, fine," Ryan said. We dropped them off and arranged a time to pick them up.

After dinner, Ryan said, "I have somewhere I want us to go."

"On a trip?" Jillian asked.

"No. Better."

They walked the length of the mall. Ryan held Jillian's hand.

"Where we going, Ryan?" she asked.

"You'll see," he said. They arrived at a jewelry store.

"Oh my God," said Jillian.

Ryan informed the clerk of his intentions: "We've been dating six years. We're very serious." Ryan introduced them. "My name is Ryan, and this is Jillian, my lovely girlfriend. I am going to marry her."

Ryan asked to see engagement rings. The clerk obliged. What the heck.

Ryan took the first diamond between his thumb and forefinger. He got down on one knee in the middle of the jewelry store in the middle of the shopping mall. "Will you make me the happiest man?" Ryan asked.

Of course, Jillian couldn't say yes fast enough. She tried on several rings, decided she preferred a thin model. "I will definitely hold on to this ring," the clerk said.

Ryan said that would be great. "I'll be coming back soon."

Soon being a relative term, of course.

Ellen once said, in the midst of one of our contrarian discussions, "Everything you've fought for is for the bigger purpose of Jillian spreading her wings. I want Jillian and Ryan to be an inspiration to other families. They're walking the front lines.

"There should be more Ryans and Jillians. There can be. Their stories can be greater than ours." Ellen imagined the evolution if kids with disabilities jumped on the Ryan-Jillian track at a far earlier age: "If they do in first grade what we didn't do until high school, who knows how this thing can evolve?"

Once when we were in the car, the big yellow taxi, I asked them why they got along so well. "You first, Ryan," I said.

"Because I love her and respect her and want to protect her," Ryan said.

"Jillian?"

"Because I trust him and have fun being with him," Jillian said.

Then they went to dinner and a movie.

CHAPTER 20

I Hope You Dance

And when you get the choice to
sit it out or dance . . .
—MARK D. SANDERS AND TIA SILLERS

On the morning of her graduation from high school, Jillian arrives in our family room, wearing a purple and white sundress and a look of expectancy. This is it. Today is May 30, 2009—her day of all days. "How do I look, Dad?" she asks.

I pull her close so she can't see the hole I'm biting into my lip. I make my eyes big because I can feel the plumbing about to burst and hope the extra room will give the water some place to go other than down my face. This is her day of triumph, not mine. "You look beautiful," I say.

"You okay, Dad?"

"Never better," I say.

I was proud of Jillian. I was proud of Kerry, who'd done 19 years of heavy hauling to get Jillian to this day. And of Kelly, whose love and support for his sister never lagged. I was proud of myself, too, in a way I could feel but not describe. It is true that the striving is the point. You do all you can, and the result will speak for itself. I was proud of myself for the daily tug, be it helping with homework or tying her shoes or pounding my fist on a conference table.

There had been lots of *Eureka!* moments in our lives with Jillian to that point. None happened without the everyday push. I was proud of the everyday push.

And it was true that I had never been better. There aren't a lot of days in our lives that truly make us feel happy for being here. Births and weddings, certainly. And graduations. Especially this graduation. To this point, everything Kerry and I had ever dreamed for Jillian, every promise we'd made to her and to each other, had come to pass. All we'd ever done for Jillian was fight for her right to be Jillian. She'd done the rest.

Graduation Day defined her. She might have other days as boldly glad as this one. All would engage the same sand and spirit she'd employed to become a high school graduate. Tears that morning honored the sand.

Kerry had picked a tune to commemorate the day. I'm always pulling lyrics from songs, wishing I could give life to feelings the way songwriters do. Van Morrison, Jackson Browne, Bruce Springsteen: All bards to me, blessed with the gift of putting essential truths to music. When Jillian was born, I played Springsteen's "Walk Like A Man" over and over. The tune isn't about a father's relationship with his daughter; it's Bruce, dealing with his feelings for his dad. No matter. I appropriated it for my own heart. A line about "steps stolen" cut especially close.

Bob Dylan informed Jillian's first days of school, each succeeding year adding to her independence and leaving Dad increasingly forlorn and melancholy. I *had* seen Jillian's ribbons and her bows, falling from her curls. Meantime, Jackson Browne told Jillian to "keep a fire burning in your eye."

And so on. Kerry wasn't as connected to this stuff as I was. She was far too practical and striving to take time to wallow in heavy-duty soul wandering. Except on this day. Kerry bought a copy of a Lee Ann Womack CD that was released nine years earlier, when Jillian was ten years old. She'd have been in third grade then.

As Jillian made her way downstairs on graduation morning, I slipped the CD's title tune into the player. "I Hope You Dance" is not complex or monumental. It speaks universal truth, though, the way lots of country songs do.

Promise me you'll give faith a fighting chance . . .

The song is about courage and preserved innocence and what Jillian would term "being my own a'vocate." It's the Jillian Daugherty Show, the two-wheeler, the homework, the dance team, the graduation Walk. *You wanna piece of me, Daddy-O?* It's possible to sum up a life in a few wonderful and corny stanzas.

I hope you never fear those mountains in the distance,
Never settle for the path of least resistance

I put my right arm across the breadth of Jillian's shoulders. My left hand slips into her right, our fingers meshing like braided rope. "Let's dance," I say.

I'd like to say the rest of the day was equally emotional. I am Irish. Blubbering at the slightest provocation comes with the sod. Van Morrison calls it the "inarticulate speech of the heart." In my heart's eye, I foresaw a pageant of tears.

I imagined Kerry and me and the healthy cast of family and friends as walking faucets. Jillian was the first child with Down syndrome ever to graduate from Loveland High School as a fully included student. The nightly Everest of homework had been scaled. The unfortunate battles with the school people had ended in an uneasy truce. Another Can-Do had been notched on Jillian Daugherty's belt. Tissues all around.

But it wasn't that way. Except for the brief dance, the day was not emotional. We never doubted that Jillian would graduate. All the striving contained an assumption that this day would come. Tears would have flowed only if she'd been derailed. It was a step, not a summit. It was cause for pride and satisfaction, no different than when Kelly graduated from the same high school five years earlier.

College was the next chapter, to be followed by a job. A life in full. High school graduation was meaningful not for the symbolism of a diploma line, but for the lessons it offered.

Jillian was atypical mainly in the lengths she went to to earn this day. We never stopped working because she never stopped trying. It was a perfect intersection of effort and courage. Giving anything less than everything we had would have been a betrayal, both of Jillian and of the ideal we had set her up to represent. We never feared those mountains in the distance.

That came with a mandate that she prove herself worthy of our pugnacious audacity. That kind of pressure might have bent a lesser kid. Jillian made it light. Jillian did the projects, wrote the papers, took the tests, earned the grades. Her papers were shorter, her tests modified to fit her abilities. The effort required was no less giant. Jillian lived up to the ideal we had created. Everest had been scaled. This was the day for planting prayer flags at the summit.

KERRY'S PARENTS WERE IN town for the occasion, as was Kerry's sister, Janis. Kerry's aunts. My brother Jeff had come from his home in Columbia, Maryland. Kelly was home from Ohio State. Nancy and Bill Croskey, and Mary Smethurst. The day would be hectically joyous. I wanted mine and Kerry's part of it to be quiet and embraceful. Before the collective roar, my daughter and I danced small circles to words of pure hope.

Whenever one door closes, I hope one more opens.

I find myself cupping the back of her head in the palm of my right hand, the same as I did when she was a few days old and her head needed supporting. We made promises to her then. She was living them now.

I asked her, as we swayed, if she understood the meaning of the words to the song. "'When you get the choice to sit it out or dance, I hope you dance.' Why is that special to you?"

Jillian, ever literal, said, "It means to be on the dance team."

"Yeah. But what else?"

"Like going to college. That's a hard thing," Jillian said. "People don't 'spect that for me."

There was one more triumph to attend to. It spoke loudly

to Jillian's impact on the people who allowed her to touch their lives. It involved a lanky six-foot-three senior named Evan Stanley.

Loveland has a tradition at its graduations. Seniors enter to "Pomp and Circumstance," two by two and do The Walk as partners to their seats. Whom you walk with is a big deal. Your partner is usually a close, longtime friend.

We worried—no, check that, I worried—that Jillian would make this next walk of a lifetime by herself. Fully included in some things, as always, but not in this thing—this essential thing. Jillian had been to Homecomings and Proms with Ryan. She'd lived those joys. She'd danced. The essential fiber of high school is not acquired in the classroom. Thirty years later, no one remembers Algebra II. What if this most social of children did this walk alone?

This was where the tide of Jillian's natural, innocence-fueled optimism met the rocks of high school reality. She was a doer, a giver and a pure heart. What she wasn't was cool. At least not as defined by her peers.

The Walk was not the same as eating alone in the cafeteria. Or never being invited to the parties typical kids threw. Those were symptoms. So was The Walk—but on a far larger scale.

"What if no one walks with her?" I asked Kerry.

"I don't know," Kerry said. She wondered, too.

As with all previous dilemmas involving Jillian's non-academic life, I didn't really want an honest answer. I wanted affirmation that someone would walk with her.

In the spring as graduation was approaching, Kerry was in the gym one day, teaching a class, when Evan Stanley walked in.

"Got a minute, Mrs. Daugherty?"

Of course. Kerry loved Evan, who befriended her daughter without reservation.

Evan paused for the briefest of moments. Kerry knew something momentous was coming.

"Would it be okay if I walked with Jillian at graduation?"

There were times when Kerry and I knew what pure joy felt like. We'd never have experienced that without Jillian. We might have thought we did. Kelly did plenty of things that made us glad to be alive. None provided the sort of life-ecstasy of Jillian's first porchlight evening. Or of Evan Stanley's simple request.

Sometimes, you want nothing more than having your kid belong. A seat at the table, a spot in the photo. We fought and fought, and we tried as hard as we could in the battles we could win. When the moments weren't so easily won, we prayed fate would be kind.

Evan didn't think what he was doing was noble or extraordinary in any way. Jillian was a real friend to him, and doing The Walk with her was logical. But he had to know that his request meant everything to us. Kerry hugged Evan and cried.

For a few weeks before graduation, Jillian spoke of nothing else.

"I'm walking at graduation with my home dog," she said.

I doubt any of Jillian's classmates knew how delighted she was about walking with Evan Stanley, her home dog. Very few of them probably gave their own walk a passing thought. They took it for granted. Jillian relished hers for weeks.

It's interesting how an extra chromosome is seen as a disability, yet its presence contributes to the sort of natural happiness Jillian possessed and shared. Evan knew that others looked at Jillian and saw Down syndrome. He saw her disability as a surface trait. "The person Jillian was, wasn't characterized by her disability," he said.

Evan was a senior at Bowling Green State in Ohio a few years later when we talked about his friendship with Jillian. They maintain a close, if infrequent, relationship. I asked him what she'd taught him.

"Don't judge a book by its cover," he said. "She taught me that, in its purest form. Having Jillian in my life definitely showed me to be open with anyone and everyone. Once you can look past what you see on the outside and the stereotypes that come with it, you can get that true friendship I think we all want and need."

Graduation was held in the 10,000-seat Cintas Center on the Xavier University campus. We sat in the upper concourse as four-foot-eight Jillian Daugherty and six-foot-three Evan Stanley made the stately walk together down the center aisle, between the rows of folding chairs, from one end of the arena floor to the

Jillian and Evan Stanley, the night of their high school graduation.

other. There have been other occasions when Jillian's peers came through when it really mattered. There still are now. None meant more than that occasion.

Jillian accepted her diploma. It was a testament to where we were emotionally that Kerry's biggest concern was how Jillian would react, center stage, upon getting that validation. Please, Jillian, no dancing. Jillian got her diploma, smiled and pumped her fist.

That's about what we did too. Sitting in the stands, I'd expected to be besieged by memories and stricken with melancholia. "Your little girl's growing up," Jillian had said to me that morning as we danced.

Instead, I was relieved. I felt we'd done our part, for Jillian and for other kids like her, younger kids, who one day would walk the same walk.

Years later, I met with Kevin Boys, the superintendent of Loveland Schools at the time Jillian graduated. I wanted to know why it had been so hard. After the race, it's easy to say how the effort was all worth it. It's harder in midstride. We never had doubts that Jillian would reach this day. We were saddened and surprised at the effort involved. Kerry and I had climbed our own Everest.

Boys was thoughtful. Far removed from his duties as superintendent—he was the president of a local college by then—Boys was candid. He said our impression that Jillian had gotten a better education early in her school years, from teachers who seemed to care more, wasn't based in fact. It came down to numbers.

"How many kids were in Jillian's second-grade class? Twenty-five? Third grade, the same. Fourth grade, the same.

Those teachers have all day to influence and teach those kids," Boys said.

"You go to middle school, you have team teaching. There are maybe five times that many kids per teacher. High school? More. You can only spread yourself so thin. We had four counselors [at Loveland High] for 1,300 kids." Boys called it "an organizational downfall of public education."

"High school teachers are different," he said. "They're much more subject-oriented than kid-oriented. [Their] job is to teach biology, not to teach kids biology."

I asked him why school officials didn't share our vision for Jillian. That had nothing to do with numbers. Why wouldn't teachers and administrators want to dream along with us? Jillian made dreaming easy. Who else loved Mondays? Sometimes, it seemed the school's mission was to hold Jillian to what it believed was the proper path instead of allowing her to blaze her own trail, just like a typical kid. How do we fix that attitude?

Boys admitted that schools "don't spend enough time on that visioning aspect. Asking ourselves, even as parents, 'What do we see our child doing', and how does this schooling" meet that vision?

"We don't have a good way to measure it. We have an IQ test. The SAT, the ACT, they predict school success, not life success. They can't judge Jillian's ability to succeed. Part of the challenge is [finding] someone who's in a position to say what a child can do. Educators can't. We don't have the tools. Parents might not be able to."

When Jillian was a sophomore, Kerry met Missy Jones. Jones was an assistant professor at Northern Kentucky University, a burgeoning commuter school 30 minutes from our house. Over the next several years, Jones would build an educational program at NKU that included people with intellectual disabilities in regular college classes with the help of student mentors.

When Kerry informed the guidance counselor at Loveland and the head of the special-education department that Jillian would be attending NKU, they each laughed dismissively. "I don't think so," they replied.

That might explain something else we found disturbing. Every copy of Jillian's Individualized Education Program included space for a parents' vision statement. Each time, Kerry included the goal of attending college. Once, when Jillian was in high school, school officials removed that paragraph from the IEP, only to reinstate it when we protested.

It is impossible to describe how it feels as a parent to be given the back of that hand. That's where our finger-jabbing comes in. Graduation day arrived on a breeze of vindication and a sigh of relief.

What if we'd listened to the school people? So many parents still listen. They allow school people to tether their children to the leash of narrow expectations, either because they don't know any better or because they're not willing to make waves. People whose careers involve furthering education for kids with intellectual disabilities claim that their biggest hurdle is not the unwillingness of schools to provide their disabled students with the basic rights to strive and dream. It is convincing parents that striving and dreaming are rights that belong to everyone, including their own special-needs children.

Jillian made the walk for herself. But the path didn't disappear. Two years after she entered NKU, her friend Sarah Klein registered for fall classes there. The Loveland schools people were excited and amazed. They took credit for Sarah's triumph. They acted as if it were their doing. Jillian was in her third year at NKU by then.

Families still threaten school districts with due process hearings to get the special services to which they are entitled. The parents of Jillian's friend Katie Daly went that route barely a year after we had. Doors opened for us. Then just as quickly closed.

"It's not that schools don't know any better," Kerry says now. "It's that schools will continue to find the cheapest way to educate."

Jillian learned to persevere because that's what she needed when she started every race with a bowling ball on her ankle. She didn't settle for the path of least resistance.

Kerry and I learned what it meant to persevere, too. We got it from Jillian.

The passage of time shivers our knees. Graduation day gets us all, in one jelly spot or another. With Jillian, it was a joy, a wonder, a pain, a pleasure, infinite sadness, timeless hope. A patience with some, a fight with others, a full-time yearn that, someday, everyone will not simply look at her, but will see her as well.

Maybe beginning today. Graduation Day.

The seas part. The world stills. She flips the tassel.

Jillian had a party that night. Kelly came with his girlfriend, Ruby. The aunts, my brother, Kerry's cousin, the grandparents Sid and Jean. Jillian's boyfriend, Ryan, and all their friends. Bill and Nancy Croskey. Evan and the homeys.

Kerry and I gathered in the middle of it all. Later on, the skies would blacken and roil. A thunderous storm sent the party indoors. For now, the night was perfectly soft. We held each other tight amid the happy chaos. "We did it," she said.

We watched our high school graduate, happy and poised and lovely, possessed of an unmistakable spirit and a warrior's heart. She stood on the back deck of our house, swaying with Ryan. They danced.

CHAPTER 21

Missy and Tommy

Jillian is Tom's legacy.
—MISSY JONES

Somehow, we remained naïve, after all the years. We operated on assumptions of optimism. Anything less would have been self-defeating. We believed the world wanted for Jillian the same things we did, even as that wasn't often so. The world wasn't always ready for us. Mostly, we earned our optimism with our sleeves rolled up. We assumed Jillian would attend college. We assumed it would be in a typical classroom setting. That's how it had worked in high school. Even with the monumental hassles, Jillian got a fully included education. Why would it be any different in college, where the intellects were keener, attitudes more forward leaning and the respect for learning more profound?

When Jillian was a sophomore at Loveland, Kerry and Ellen went to Columbus to attend a national Down syndrome conference on postsecondary education for students with cognitive disabilities. Ryan was a year ahead of Jillian in school so Ellen's interest was especially pressing. Like Kerry and me, Ellen believed the college experience would be easier and more pleasurable for everyone.

We had begun a college fund for Jillian when she was born, just as we had for Kelly. We'd included college in all the IEP vision statements. We'd made it through her high school graduation without backstroking through our tears because we considered graduation to be the next brick in the wall. Kerry went to Columbus invested in all those notions but was entirely taken aback by what she saw when she got there.

Colleges had "programs" in which students with intellectual disabilities were assigned to their own rooms on campus. They would learn "life skills." Someone would teach them how to make their beds, do their laundry and use public transportation. The schools would offer them menial campus jobs. Apparently, they thought this was cutting edge, and they were proud of it.

Once Jillian was tall enough to reach the knobs on the washer and dryer, she was washing her own clothes. She made her bed and her own meals. She didn't need a "program" for that. She needed a typical college experience that would involve her taking actual classes and making actual rounds of the campus. We saw no benefit in her being sequestered in a classroom of kids just like her, learning to make a perfect square corner with a bedsheet.

We posed the same questions we'd asked more than a decade earlier: If you want a student to learn to speak, do you put him in a classroom full of mutes? If your child has behavioral issues, would you like to see him with a roomful of kids acting out? What's being reinforced there?

"It wasn't quite what we were looking for," Kerry said.

She could not have been more disappointed. The world wasn't opening up. It seemed to be offering a new set of doors. The only way to discover what was beyond them was to roll up our sleeves again, this time to the shoulders. Optimism is mandatory, and exhausting.

At lunch in a big banquet hall on the Ohio State University campus, Kerry and Ellen traded lamentations. They sounded like this: "Can you believe what they thought was a college education? If we want our kids to learn how to make their beds, we'll teach them. We don't need to pay a college for that."

There were a couple thousand conference-goers positioned at round, linen-draped tables for 12. Kerry and Ellen began commiserating with their table-mates, all strangers. Then something wonderful happened. I called it serendipitous, even though I am not a big believer in serendipity. Things happen for a reason. Fate is a spectator, not a participant. And yet I have seen some serendipitous things in Jillian's life. Moments that couldn't be explained. Seemingly random acts of benevolent coincidence have swayed me toward some belief in a greater hand, unseen.

Missy Jones just happened to be seated across the table from Kerry and Ellen. She was an assistant professor at Northern Kentucky University. She was as committed as Kerry and Ellen when it came to inclusive education. Missy heard every word Kerry and Ellen were saying.

"They were disappointed. I was energized," Missy recalled.

It had all begun at Missy's home some 50 years earlier.

Stars always align in some fashion. The talent is in seeing the good in every alignment.

It was hard to see any good on that day in 1954, when Tommy Thompson was born with the umbilical cord wrapped around his neck. It had been in that position, denying his brain oxygen, for the better part of a week before his arrival. Tommy was a "blue baby." Doctors delivered him, then resuscitated him. He was Missy Jones's older brother by five years. Her story begins with him.

Tommy entered the world with mild cerebral palsy. The left side of his brain was damaged, so he never had full use of the right side of his body. Doctors told Jim and Marge Thompson their son would never walk. As Marge recalled, they suggested that "Someday, you'll want to put him in an institution."

Jillian's story lacks that sort of medieval thinking. That doesn't mean it's entirely dissimilar. Jillian is who Tommy might have been, had he been given the opportunities she has had.

The Thompsons wouldn't hear any of the advice they were being given. "He's my son," Marge said simply.

The Thompsons practiced inclusion, as least as it was defined in the 1960s. They included Tommy in everything they did. Society gave them only so much rope though. "Back then, you hid your kids" with disabilities, Marge Thompson said.

Tommy played with other neighborhood kids. He went everywhere his family went: On vacations, out to eat, to the country club where Jim played golf. Tommy drove Jim's cart. They held their son to the same standard as their daughters. He cleaned his room, did the dishes, cut the grass. If he misbehaved, he was punished. "If we treated him differently, he would have acted differently," Marge explained.

The Thompsons moved around the country as Jim chased his career dreams. Eventually, they landed in Cincinnati. At every stop, Marge would enroll Missy and her two sisters in school. She'd also ask about Tommy. None of the typical schools would let Tommy attend. There were places he could go, segregated schools and sheltered workshops. At the workshops, Tommy would perform menial tasks such as assembling cardboard boxes until there were none left to be done. Then he would be ordered to put his head on the table and be silent the rest of the day. That could be hours, just sitting there, with his head on a table.

At one point, Marge pulled Tommy from a workshop where he sat idle most of the day. He never went back. No one from the workshop ever called to ask where he'd gone.

Tommy, like Jillian, had an innate compassion that captivated his family. Missy would arrive home on the school bus from kindergarten, and there would be her big brother, ten years old, sitting on a rock at the end of the driveway, waiting for her. Jillian had her rock, too, where she sat and waved goodbye to her brother and his friends on Saturday nights.

As Missy got older, on the rare occasions when she had friends over, she would never tell them about her brother's condition. She wanted to see how they'd react upon meeting him. The responses ran the spectrum from fear to disdain to compassion and complete comfort. Missy called her brother "my thermometer on the world." I remember that Kelly never kept friends who didn't also embrace his sister.

When Missy learned to drive a car with a manual transmission, Tommy sat in the passenger seat, shifting the gears as she worked the clutch. Decades later, Jillian would ride in my lap, steering my car down empty country roads, insisting she could drive.

Jillian has expanded the possibilities. Tommy would have liked her. It's not that Jillian has more innate ability than Tommy. But she has been given more opportunity and experienced more. The world's classroom is no longer so segregated.

Jim Thompson owned two Orange Julius franchises at local shopping malls. Tommy worked at one and became accomplished at squeezing oranges, making soft pretzels and washing towels. Given a purpose and some responsibility, Tommy thrived. He lived at home, worked, cut the grass, washed dishes, and did his laundry. He had a full life.

Shortly after getting her doctorate, Missy began teaching a graduate course in special education at NKU. One of her students was a special-ed teacher at a local high school who was looking for ways to "meaningfully include" her intellectually disabled students in some sort of college experience. Missy started by giving extra credit to her grad students for taking these high school kids to lunch.

She was surprised to learn that parents wanted more for their kids than the occasional social outing or campus job. During focus groups, Missy heard parents advocate for a typical college experience that included classroom work. It was an epiphany for Missy, who also wondered why these kids couldn't take regular classes like everyone else.

This was about the time she attended the conference in Columbus and overheard Kerry and Ellen at lunch. "I'd like to introduce myself," Missy said.

Kerry started the morning dispirited and ended the day enriched. She learned what she didn't want for Jillian. And she met Missy Jones, someone who thought the way she did. After living a vagabond life growing up, she had now settled in suburban Cincinnati. As soon as Missy launched her program, we wanted Jillian to be a part of it.

In 2012, NKU was one of two universities in the country that had a fully included program for students with intellectual disabilities.

Was this fate? I don't know. I think about it, just as Galileo pondered the alignment of the stars. It's about as knowable.

I see the chances Jillian has been given and what she has made of them. I know only this: None of us is in this alone. We all need a few hands to help tug our lives. Whether they arrive by design or fate or something greater and more cosmic, we'll never know. All we can do is use all that is given to us to the fullest.

Fate and need had bisected opportunity at a sweet spot in time. Ryan Mavriplis enrolled at NKU in the fall of 2008 as part of Missy's nascent program. Jillian Daugherty followed him a year later.

By 2011, 27 colleges were getting federal grant money. Some remained entirely segregated. They were what Missy called "Special-Ed College." Others were hybrids that allowed students to take two "typical" classes while also getting the life skills indoctrination. Missy believes only two universities in the country remain fully included, one being NKU.

Marge Thompson raised Tommy at home. Thanks to his family, he was the best he could be. Thanks to Tommy, his family learned some things about the beauty of difference. That said, Marge never thought that her son could ever have lived even remotely independently. "She couldn't envision taking it as far as we have," Missy said.

Walls to bridges. Jillian has never been anchored to the low expectations presented to Tommy in the 1960s. His dreams then would be Jillian's nightmares now. And yet, their goals are the same. Dignity. Respect. A place where they can hold their heads up and belong.

Jillian fights to be seen and not looked at. That's a world of difference from Tommy Thompson. It didn't occur to the world that he was worth seeing.

Sadly, Tommy didn't live long enough to see the world for people with disabilities change for the better. In 1984, Marge Thompson heard her son coughing violently in his bedroom. "Are you going to throw up?" she asked.

Tommy leaned over his bed, practically doubled over, trying to vomit. He sat back up, still coughing. Marge ran to the telephone in the hallway, just outside Tommy's door, and called an ambulance. "My son is dying," she said.

She went back into his room long enough for him to look at her, take a breath and close his eyes.

The autopsy revealed that Tommy Thompson had died of a pulmonary edema. He was 29 years old. The coroner later said that on average three people a year in the Cincinnati area died the same way, usually at about age 30. Their lungs fill with fluid, and they choke to death.

Tommy's death had nothing to do with his disability. It just happened.

After Tommy died, Missy and her two sisters went their separate ways. One lives in Cleveland, the other in Arizona. Marge Thompson is 84 years old and lives with Missy in Cincinnati.

A few times a day now, Jillian, Ryan or any of the other students in the program will pop into Missy Jones's office. They just chat, mostly. If they have a problem with a class or one of their mentors, maybe they'll bring that up. Usually, they just enjoy the fellowship.

I asked Missy about Tommy's legacy. She takes a long look at the photographs on her office wall. There are some of Tommy at his segregated school, doing his best, being Tommy.

"Jillian," she said. "Jillian is Tom's legacy. Ryan is his legacy. Anyone who is having an opportunity to reach out and experience life to its fullest is his legacy. It's my parents' legacy, too, whether they know it or not."

Tommy Thompson is buried in Cincinnati, right next to his dad. We can't know how life would have been different for him had he been born 35 years later. Or maybe we can. She's right there, standing in Missy Jones's office doorway. The Jillian Daugherty Show, just passing by on her way to class, wanting to say hello.

CHAPTER 22

College

*If you're alive to the possibility of what's different,
it gives you a gift every time you go. You can play
bad. You can make a lousy score. But you
can't lose. And I love that.*
—BILL CLINTON, *GOLF DIGEST*, FEBRUARY 2012

On an impossibly bright morning in September 2009, Jillian ker-bumped from the passenger seat of the family taxi and stepped into her newest future. High school graduation hadn't been the end of the school bus line for her. It was a transfer stop. They called it "commencement." A beginning. Yes.

The accoutrements were the same: An impossibly fat 30-pound green backpack, a first-day hairdo—short and neat, parted to one side—and the familiar happy-hop in her step that telegraphs both Jillian's mood and her presence.

But everything was different. This was a new frontier. It was an unfamiliar rung on the ladder of possibility. It was Jillian's first day of college.

"I'm having a great day so far," she announced on the short drive from our home to the campus of Northern Kentucky University. It was barely 9:00 a.m. Jillian spent most of the ride staring intently at four index cards Kerry had made for her first day. They contained basic information: The names and places of her two classes; how to get from the car to the elevator of the BPE building, what button to push, where to go from there. Jillian read them over and over even though she'd done a trial run a few days earlier.

"When I get on the elevator, I go to the second floor," Jillian announced.

"Yes," I said.

She also had a form that allowed her to use a digital recorder to tape the lectures. Jillian will ask another student to take notes for her. They will supplement Jillian's own notes. Missy Jones will appoint a mentor to help Jillian with her work and getting socialized.

She will take two classes, American History Since 1865 and University 101, an introduction to NKU all students must take. Between the mentor, the note taker, the tape recorder and Jillian's own efforts, we will scale this newest hill. Sometimes at a sprint, sometimes while running in place. Always ready should the wheels come off.

I don't recall what I expected of that day specifically, or of the thousand or so since. You can have high expectations without being specific. General goals are flexible and more easily adjusted. I know I wanted the same for Jillian that day that

I wanted for all of her first days: Do your best. Be your best. Seize the moment. Be Jillian.

I was afraid, though. For every other milestone, we'd held Jillian's hand, sometimes literally. If we weren't at school, we were a ten-minute drive away. Public secondary school was a leap, but within a self-contained environment. One building, all day, cocooned by any number of teachers and peers, most of whom knew her, and she them. Jillian's newest future was on 400 acres, with more than 40 buildings, filled with 13,000 undergrads. This big, sprawling room of possibility didn't know my daughter.

During the previous year, when she was a senior in high school, we drove Jillian to NKU four times, twice in February and twice more in April. She took an orientation tour of the campus, observed classes and met potential mentors. Twice during the summer, after Jillian had gotten her schedule, Kerry walked her to her classrooms.

Kerry also made sure Jillian's college experience included things a typical college student would need if she were going away to school. Jillian and Kerry went shopping for new comforters and pillows and towels, as if Jillian would be moving into a dorm room. The preparation had been thorough. Jillian was as ready for college as all of us could make her. What of the expectations?

I had a vague notion of what I wanted college to be for her. I wasn't silly enough to think Jillian would learn the way a typical college student would. She had graduated from high school mostly because she'd met all the requirements, not because she was as adept at her schoolwork as even the lowest-achieving typical child.

College would accelerate that. Jillian would do what she'd done in high school: Learn at her pace, with help. Work as hard as anyone. She wouldn't get a degree. She was registered as a non–degree-seeking student. But that didn't mean she wouldn't get an education. It didn't mean she wouldn't learn. I wanted Jillian to learn more how to belong, how to get along. It would be a social experiment as much as anything. I wanted her to cope with her disability in a wider world. I wanted her to sing her triumphs to a broader audience, one older and wiser enough to see her for who she was, not who she wasn't.

I wanted all this in the larger landscape beyond one building and seven bells a day. I wanted her to have friendships. Not superficial, patronizing acquaintances, but relationships, deep and impactful. I wanted people to feel better for having known her. I wanted them to understand that learning defies shapes and sizes and boundaries. We're all lifetime learners.

As much as I wanted Jillian to be taught, I wanted her to teach.

There was an implied contract I wanted satisfied. I wanted NKU to be open-minded and big-hearted. I wanted Jillian embraced in a way she never was in high school, and I wanted it because it was the right and enlightened thing to do.

I wanted her to come to the party bearing gifts, not just receiving them. I believed she would emerge more independent and more self-assured, in the way all adults should be. I wanted her time at NKU to be joyous and responsible and fulfilling. I wanted her to leave there purposeful and confident, and happy for the time she'd spent. I wanted everyone she met to feel the same.

I wanted all that from her very first day. I had no idea if any of it would happen.

There was a model, though. There was a precedent. A few years earlier, I had met Deb Hart. Hart is the director of education and transition at the Institute for Community Inclusion at UMass-Boston. That is a big title for someone who is basically a grassroots battler. Hart has spent 40 years plowing the hard and dry fields of Why-Not. She can tell you about perceptions and stereotypes and the act of moving a mountain. "It's very hard for humans to change," she says.

Hart began her work in 1973, 16 years before Jillian was born, as a student teacher in the Massachusetts public schools. We forget now what it was like in 1973 to be someone like Jillian or Ryan. Deb Hart recalls it vividly. Much of her work involved changing hearts and minds, and not just those within the school and governmental bureaucracies. Parents also needed educating. "You have to have high expectations," she said.

PARENTS SHARED IN THE low expectations. Part of the problem was that nobody had ever told them their kids could learn. Nobody ever offered them a Why-Not. From the maternity ward to the public schools, parents had been told their kids with special needs could not achieve.

Parents also had grown comfortable with the babysitting approach to special education. It's safe and easy. Parents welcome the extra four years of high school that the law allows. They want the benefits that accrue from not working.

"They've had to fight for benefits. The thought of something that's going to mess with that" doesn't appeal to them, Hart said. "To get Social Security benefits you have to show you can't work. Our special education system has had the un-intended consequence of enabling dependence. It encourages students with disabilities to be satisfied. Their families didn't teach independent living skills, so special ed did."

Into this evolving landscape marched Jillian Daugherty. We arrived at the drop-off area, and Jillian looked up from her notes. "This is it, Dad," she said. "I'm a little bit nervous, a little bit."

"Everybody's nervous on their first day," I said. "You have your phone and your directions?"

"Yes, Dad."

"Lunch?"

"Yep."

I told her everything would be fine. I said it more for my benefit than Jillian's. Assuring Jillian that college would be fine was like lecturing a mouse on the possibilities in 300 pounds of cheese. Even if she was nervous, a little bit.

"You're good, right?" I asked. So lame.

"Yes, Dad."

I squeezed her hand as she exited the car. "I can't tell you how proud we are of you," I say. "I love you very much. What a great day. Have fun."

"Okay, Dad," Jillian says.

I told her I'd wait in the lot a few minutes. "Call if you need help," I said

"Don't worry 'bout it," Jillian answered. "Your little girl is in college now."

And there she went.

CHAPTER 23

In the Swing

*I am not concerned that you have fallen—I am
concerned that you arise.*
—ABRAHAM LINCOLN

We picked her up at 2:30 p.m. in the same place I'd dropped her off. We didn't know what to expect. We should have though. Just because Kerry and I had been fearful didn't mean Jillian would be. And she wasn't.

"My history teacher, oh my God, he makes me laugh," she said the minute she got in the backseat.

"So, you had a good day?"

"Yeah. You guys, it was the best," Jillian said.

That wasn't exactly true. It was Jillian, spinning the moment to fit her personality.

In her second class, the professor suggested a getting-to-know-you game. The students stood, declared their names, then offered an alliterative description of themselves.

I'm Rob, and I'm romantic. I'm Melissa who's money-conscious.

Jillian jumped up at her appointed moment. "I'm Jillian, and I like to eat."

"Okay, this is Jillian who likes to read," the professor said, misunderstanding Jillian's words.

"She doesn't understand me," Jillian said of the professor later, at home. She seemed a little overwhelmed. "I don't know anyone," she said.

"It was your first day, sweets," I said. "Everybody feels a little weird their first day of college." I meant what I said. I wasn't sure I believed it in Jillian's case. Her college experience would be as new to me as it was to her.

Jillian spent a few hours after that writing manically in her journal. It was a written version of the Jillian Daugherty Show. There were names of people she met, what her professors said, how she navigated successfully from classroom to Student Union, back to classroom. And this, the last sentence of the entry: "My parents are proud of their college girl."

We were just getting warmed up.

Calling what was happening to Jillian a "college experience" explains everything and nothing. No two are quite alike. When someone says he had a good experience in college, I picture fraternity debauchery and Southern Comfort at football games. Kerry laments that part of my existence. "I wouldn't have liked you when you were in college," she says.

Where I went to school, it was not an expellable offense to set ablaze a rival frat's grand piano and roll it down the center of the street. I attended an all-male college surrounded by five women's colleges, each conveniently located within an hour's drive. We misbehaved at our leisure on weekdays. On weekends, we took it seriously.

Kerry went to school to get her degree. She was on the dance team. She was a straight-arrow student. I wouldn't have liked her either when she was in college.

We convened on the back deck after Jillian's first day to share our impressions. I asked Kerry what she wanted Jillian to take from NKU. She said "a typical college experience."

I said if she got anywhere near a fraternity house, I would lock her in her room for four years straight.

"I want her to take academic classes," Kerry corrected. "I want her walking the campus, being part of a community."

We could have driven Jillian to class and killed time until she finished, then picked her up. Instead, we dropped her off in time for her 10:00 a.m. class and picked her up late in the afternoon. We encouraged her to discover the campus. To fill the in-between hours, Jillian had to be engaged and resourceful.

She ate lunch in the Student Union, often going through the buffet line. She found a place with wireless and used her laptop to surf the Net. She took gym clothes and worked out in the Health Center. She needed to mind the time, to be where she needed to be. This is what Kerry meant by a "college experience." Jillian was getting her wings. We wanted her to fly as far as she could.

Some parents were incredulous that we would set Jillian free that way. They said we were setting her up to fail. They missed the point. We did want Jillian to fail.

Not entirely, of course. Every day of that first year I worried that Jillian would become lost and confused and scared.

I worried that someone on campus would take advantage of her kindness and innocence. Jillian believes everyone is good. That's nice, in a conceptual kind of way, but scary on a wide-open campus of 13,000 students.

But everyday, small-scale failure was okay.

"That's how we learn," Kerry said that first day. "I hope Jillian gets lost. I want her to get lost. I want things to go wrong. Then I want her to figure them out and make them right."

We weren't raising Jillian to stay with us. We were raising her to leave. Same as her brother. This was the next step.

It turns out she did get lost. Missy Jones would e-mail Kerry occasionally to say that Jillian was in the wrong building. Missy offered to appoint a student to walk Jillian to class, but we said no. Jillian had a cell phone and a campus full of peers. She had her index cards. She could call someone or ask for help. She can cope. That's part of why she's there.

And so she did. Soon enough, Jillian stopped getting lost. She never called Kerry or me for help. She had no escorts. She started enjoying her time on campus and away from us. She had her favorite places. She ate lunch with Ryan, she ran on the treadmill at the Health Center. She asked to be picked up later in the day. "I love my school," she said daily.

It changed her in other ways too. Jillian became more independent, which meant she needed us less. Her developmental delays had extended to her attitude. The Parents Are Gross era that most kids experience in intermediate school and high school came on for Jillian as a college student. "How was your day?" would be answered with "Good."

"What did you do? Tell me everything," I might say. To

which Jillian would respond, "Dad, I'm a college student now. I do lots of things."

Well, okay. We were put off by her responses but pleased at the independence they described.

Jillian knows she isn't like everyone else. But at school, she feels she is. She's part of the universal to-and-from, the easy here-and-there that defines college life. She has a backpack, an iPod and a Mac. She has a purse and an All-Card for student activities and a key card that gets her into the gym. She uses the same books everyone else does. She's a manager on the basketball team, too, a duty that occupies two hours a day, five days a week, not including games.

There was another piece to the independence puzzle though. Jillian needed to learn to get from A to B without us. NKU was essentially a commuter school. Its typical students drove or took the bus to campus. Jillian had to learn to use public transportation.

Transportation is freedom. Freedom is independence. Independence is what we're working toward here. If Jillian and Ryan could manage public transportation, they could get places on their own. It would let them get to the grocery store, the mall, the movies—and eventually from their own apartment to the essentials and the pleasures of the day to day.

We started this next grand experiment the second semester of Jillian's second year at NKU. Initially, the plan was for Jillian to take the bus to NKU only. We'd pick her up after school. In the mornings, I would drive Jillian to the Metro stop closest to our house, getting her there in time to catch an

8:05 a.m. bus to downtown Cincinnati. From there, she would transfer to another bus that would get her to school.

Step two involved the reverse: NKU to home.

First, we made a dry run. I met Jillian and Ryan on campus on a blustery day in January.

The Number 11 TANK (Transportation Authority of Northern Kentucky) bus leaves the NKU campus at 2:01 p.m. "Not 2:00," I tell Ryan and Jillian. "Not 2:02." The inference was, Be on time. Not as freighted with worldly concerns as the rest of us, Ryan and Jillian tend to float. They don't take straight lines to places. They prefer the winding road. The scenery's better.

"If you're late, the bus leaves without you."

"Yes, sir," Ryan says.

This was a big day in their lives. It was heavy with symbolism. Get up in the morning, get on the bus. Go to work. Produce. Enter the land of the meaningful. Feel you belong and act on the feeling. Get on the bus.

I tell Jillian and Ryan to be at the bus stop at 1:50 p.m. They get there at 1:50 p.m., fresh from class, holding hands, smiling, ready. They want to know everything. Will it stop right here? Do I need money? How do I know when I'm finished? That's what Jillian asked: "How do I know when I'm finished?"

"Listen to me," I say.

"Yes, sir," Ryan says.

Jillian has a fistful of bus schedules and her student ID that will allow her to ride for free on the first leg of the journey, the eight miles from NKU to downtown Cincinnati. For the second leg, which will cost $2.65, she has packed a Zip-Loc sandwich bag full of quarters. The bag must hold 40 quarters.

I tell Ryan the first bus is free with his ID card. "I have this," he says, fishing through his wallet. He pulls out a card that is good for a free bowl of soup. "Keep looking," I say.

I will ride with them. I will tell them when to get off the first bus and where to get on and off the second bus. I'll tell them what it costs. I'll help them to slide the dollar bills into the money box: "Flat. President Washington's head pointing this way, like the diagram."

"See?"

"Yes, sir."

I will show them the marquee attached to the ceiling at the front of the bus. It runs continuously, a stream of information, like a sports crawl across the bottom of an ESPN channel: Bus name, bus destination, time of day. I will tell them when the bus is scheduled to arrive at its destination. "Look at the time up there," I say to them. "When that time gets close to the time you're supposed to get off, start paying attention."

They nod.

I show Ryan the cord above his head. "You pull that when you want to get off," I say.

"Got it," he says.

The first bus arrives precisely at 2:01 p.m. "See?" I say. "Right on time. You guys need to be prompt when you take the bus. Do you know what prompt means?"

"I think so," Jillian says. "What?"

"It means be here exactly when you're supposed to be," I say.

"Exactly," says Jillian.

Ryan says, "Yes, sir."

The inside of a city bus isn't the likeliest place to discover wonder or contentment. It's all about poker faces and gum beneath the seats. Unless you are Jillian and Ryan, who find wonder in just about everything. The bus moves slowly, circuitously and with frequent stops. Ryan and Jillian can relate. Ryan reads aloud the sign that hangs above the seats closest to the doors: "Please allow seniors and persons with disabilities to use these seats when requested."

"You guys wanna move up there?" I ask.

"I'm comfy here," Jillian says.

They've been together a lifetime, or so it seems. They are people who enjoy each other's company and have for more than five years. I know adults married five years who can't stand the sight of each other. We all do. Jillian and Ryan are an old married couple. I'm comfy here, she says.

The bus passes a dance studio. Jillian notices the sign above the studio door. "I think we should do ballroom dancing again," she announces. They'd taken a class together a few years earlier, a Christmas present to each other.

"I do not want to do ballroom dancing," Ryan says. It's midday. The bus is not crowded: A couple of students, a day laborer in gray overalls, released from his morning shift. Jillian, Ryan and me.

"I love your daughter, and I will always take care of her," Ryan says, just because the thought occurred.

"I'm happy about that," I say.

The bus chugs haltingly, stop to stop. It's not the most efficient method of traveling, but it does give Ryan time to be social. Passengers come and go. Ryan makes them feel important. "Have a good day, sir," he says to the guy in the overalls. The man looks up, a little wide-eyed. Maybe no one ever wished him well on the bus before. "Bless you," Ryan says.

The rocking and swaying is making him drowsy. "You can't fall asleep," I tell Ryan.

"We can't?"

"Nope. You could sleep right through your stop."

I suggest that one person could sleep, so long as the other is awake. Jillian and Ryan think that's a good idea. Especially Ryan. "Wake me up, honey," he says.

Everything is new. When he's awake, Ryan reads every word on the inside of the bus. He hears the computerized voice announce upcoming stops. "Who's talking?" he wonders. Jillian checks out the storefronts. The pizza joints, the dance studio, the restaurants and the sports bars, especially the sports bars, with their neon signs in the windows.

"Ryan, you can get a beer there," Jillian says.

"Cool," says Ryan.

The TANK bus crosses the Ohio River and moves on into downtown Cincinnati. The nest of streets thickens, there are more people, and the pace speeds exponentially. Jillian and Ryan's eyes get a little bigger. They're suburban kids.

"This is downtown Cincinnati?" Jillian asks.

"Yes."

"Where your office is?"

"Yes." Well, sort of. I work at home or at the ballpark or arena. My newspaper building is downtown.

Ryan knows we're getting close. He reaches his arm toward the stop cord. "You don't want to pull that yet," I say.

"When?"

"I'll tell you."

"Yes, sir."

The bus nears Fourth and Main, their stop. I tell Ryan to pull the cord. We get out, but not where I think we're supposed to. I had assumed the bus would stop at the large downtown terminal. Instead, it stops a block south. We have 12 minutes to find the stop for the Number 3X bus, the one to Kenwood.

I'm confused. The schedule says the 3X picks up at Fourth and Main, right where the 11 bus left us off. But the sign there makes no mention of the 3X bus. We walk up the block, to the left, toward the terminal.

This is where I should mention that I am the one who's lost. The leader of the pack, the adult, the guide: Lost. Jillian and Ryan are following me, and I have no idea what I'm doing.

"Hang on a minute," I say.

Oh. It also might be worth noting that when we boarded the bus at NKU, I had to borrow money from my daughter. I had only a $10 bill; the fare was $1.75. Exact change only, please.

When we boarded the second bus, I had to borrow more. I guess I needed my own Zip-Loc bag of quarters. Also, in the midst of note taking about this trip, my pen ran out of ink. What is it we say about people who have Down syndrome and people who don't? We're more alike than different?

"Jills, you got a pen I can borrow?" I ask.

She does. We're only as good as the way we treat each other. I wouldn't have been able to ride the bus or write what I saw. Not without my responsible, prepared and forward-thinking kid. The one with Down syndrome.

We trudge on, toward the terminal on Fifth Street. It is January. A light rain falls in the 40-degree bluster. We get to the big terminal, three lanes across, several shelters. There are signs for seemingly every bus route in and around Cincinnati. I read every one of them. I ask Jillian and Ryan to do the same. There is no 3X bus to Kenwood. There is a kiosk at one end of the terminal. I ask the man inside about the 3X bus.

"Sixth Street, a block up," he says.

"Yeah, but the schedule says Fourth," I say.

"Sixth, Fourth, either one," he says.

"Okay, but I didn't see a sign for the 3X bus at Fourth and Main," I say.

I'm sounding a little panicked—six minutes before the bus comes!—and overall pathetic. The guy behind the glass owns the weary look of someone whose life is too full of people asking stupid, pleading questions.

"Walgreen's," he says.

What? By now, I'm losing what little patience for myself I have left. The temperature is 40 degrees and it's raining. With me are two young adults who trust me to know what I'm doing, and now we're down to five minutes before the 3X bus departs and leaves us freezing on a downtown street.

"The stop you want is in front of Walgreen's, okay?" the guy says.

Having already revealed my naked ineptitude, I don't dare ask him where, exactly, the Walgreen's is on Fourth Street.

Jillian and Ryan stand quietly behind me, shivering in the mist. They've taken their backpacks from their backs. They're looking a little solemn. "We lost, Dad?" Jillian asks.

"We got it now," I reply. "We're straight."

This was good, actually, I tell them, as we head around the block toward the holy land of Walgreen's and, please God, the stop for the 3X bus. "This is what you do when you don't know something. You ask," I say. "This was a good lesson in problem solving."

We're all but running—I at a brisk walk, the two of them at a steady trot. These are small people, with small legs. Ryan is just over five feet, Jillian six inches beneath him. My incompetence is forcing them to run in the cold rain.

"Gotta go, gotta go," I say.

"This is fun," Ryan says.

God bless him.

We make the corner, left from Fifth to Fourth. We are back where we started. Three minutes before the bus is supposed to arrive at 2:53 p.m. And there it is! Walgreen's is up a block, across the street, maybe 50 paces from where we got off the TANK bus.

"We had 'em all the way," I say.

Jillian says, "What?"

We stand briefly in the rain at Fourth Street and Vine, waiting for the 3X. A newspaper box containing a free weekly catches Ryan's eye. "You should read that. It tells you places where you can take your girlfriend for a hot night on the town," I suggest.

"Ooooh," Jillian says. "I like a hot town."

The ride from downtown to suburbia is 15 miles. It takes 55 minutes. The bus stops and fills every other corner. The riders wear empty expressions, neither good nor bad. It's just part of the drill. Jillian rests her head on Ryan's shoulder. The gentle swaying of the bus would put anyone to sleep. She closes her eyes. "My eyes are open, sir," Ryan says.

The journey ends in Kenwood, a well-off suburb. The stop is across a busy street from an upscale shopping mall, filled with sit-down restaurants. Jillian and Ryan exit the bus, hand-in-hand. She has already made plans for the next bus ride.

"Ryan," she says excitedly. "Cheesecake Factory."

CHAPTER 24

Sometimes, We Drove

They have all these places for lunch.
—JILLIAN

As much as I wanted Jillian to ride the bus, I missed the time we had in the car during her first year in college. Three days a week, we'd pile in, semi-awake. I'd pick up Ryan and away we'd go. Thirty minutes doesn't sound like a lot of time, but you can learn a lot in half an hour.

"Top o' the mornin' to ye," I'd say, when Ryan got in the car.

"Top o' the mornin', sir," he'd say. And away we went.

Somedays, Jillian and Ryan would sit in the backseat together. Others, for reasons unknown, at least to the driver, Jillian rode shotgun. On this particular day, Ryan has the backseat to himself. He leans forward and starts massaging his girlfriend's shoulders. "I take good care of your daughter, sir," he says.

"I know you do."

"Honey?" Ryan says.

Jillian has fallen asleep. I nudge her awake. "Your man is talking to you."

"Yeah, Ryan?"

"Do you like this?" Ryan asks, his fingers busy across the tops of Jillian's shoulders.

Jillian says she does.

"When we get married, I will do this every night," Ryan says.

"We not ready yet," Jillian says. She will be 20 in a month. Ryan is all of 22.

"Aw, honey." Ryan is protesting from the backseat. He remembers the salesman at the mall jewelry store. "Our guy won't hold that ring forever."

Jillian says, "Ryan?" It is more a declaration than an interrogation.

"Yes?" Ryan says. His fingers are working double-time.

"You are my best boy. But I will tell you when we will get married."

I chime in. "Ryan, if you elope with my daughter, I will hunt you down."

"What does that mean, sir?"

He wants to talk about the concept of eloping. I do not.

"I will hire a pack of bloodhounds and the FBI. When they find you, I will tell them to strip you naked and feed your fingertips to the wolverines."

Ryan wants to know what a wolverine is.

Jillian says, "Da-a-a-d."

There were mornings when they discussed that evening's date—Dewey's Pizza or Mimi's Café?—and whether they'd see the newest Pixar movie or the new one with Justin Bieber.

"Parents don't do both," I'd suggest. "We save money. We do one or the other."

"We do both," Jillian said.

There were mornings when they discussed their families as if I weren't right there, driving the cab.

"My dad yelled at my brother last night," Jillian might say.

"Why, honey?"

"Somethin' 'bout money."

Ryan added that one of his brothers was grounded. "My mom was really mad," he said.

"About what?" I asked. I was curious about why Ryan and Jillian would talk about family things in front of me. And you know, I was interested in why one of Ryan's brothers was grounded.

"Sorry sir," Ryan said. "I won't talk anymore."

"You can talk, Ryan," Jillian said.

This particular morning, I started the trip by asking Jillian what she liked about college. Just about every day, she would declare that she was a big fan. On this day, I wanted to know why.

"The restaurants," she said

"I'm sorry?"

"They have all these places for lunch."

"Yeah, I know, sweetie. But what about classes? What about that great college experience you're having? You know, the whole independence, being-your-own-advocate thing. That stuff. What about that stuff?" I asked.

"They have Starbuck's," Jillian said.

She had always been a big fan of food, and that hadn't

changed. The weekend errand runs that prompted Jillian's fast-food riffs hadn't ended. They'd simply shifted locales. For some of us, dining out is a big sucking sound in the right rear pants pocket. To Jillian, it is a basic human need.

"Sushi," Jillian said.

"What?"

"I eat sushi for lunch sometimes."

"Nobody eats sushi for lunch," I said. "Especially not college kids. Especially not this college kid, whose parents are paying tuition and for her lunch."

"I eat sushi," said Jillian. "I love sushi."

The student union at NKU is food heaven. Seemingly every eatery of her youth has gathered for a convention, right in the middle of campus. This thrills her. Jillian's best college experience, evidently, is choosing between tacos and fried wontons. I draw the line, however, at sushi. "No sushi for lunch," I said to my daughter the college gourmand. "Got it?"

"Okay," she said. "Chef salad."

Whatever.

"Let's change the subject," I offered. "How are your classes?"

"I love my acting class," Jillian said. "I'll show you guys tonight."

"Can't wait," I said innocently.

For her first year at NKU, we'd decided to split Jillian's classes between core courses and electives. She took Dance and Public Speaking one semester, Spanish and Acting the next. The Jillian Daugherty show played well within the confines of Drama 101. That night, we got a brief performance. Jillian bopped around the family room, pointing fingers and pretending to drink a beer. Her professor had asked her to produce a scene with which she was familiar. Uh-oh.

"Oh, my God," she said. Jillian held her head with both hands. "I can't believe it. I just drank six beers."

"Wait," I said to Kerry. "I thought I said no fraternities in the college experience!"

Jillian was in a bar. At least this is what she said. It could be a gentlemen's club, as she was making references to women in cages.

"Bartender!" my 19-year-old daughter yelled. "Another round!"

Because she operates in a guileless, agenda-free world, this is either acting in its purest form, or it's not acting at all. We guessed an acting class would be a natural for Jillian. We were right. Whether that's good or bad we'd begun to wonder.

"Hey, baby," Jillian said.

Baby?

She was talking with a man in the bar. I could feel the crimp on my face spreading across my eyes and a frown at the corners of my mouth. "Um, Jillian . . ."

"No, no, Dad. Wait," she said.

"Do you want a beer?" she asked.

"Watching this, yeah, absolutely," I said. "Maybe more than one."

"No, Dad. I'm acting."

"Oh."

"What's your name?" Jillian asked the bar patron.

"What the . . ."

"Dad. Dad. Stop. Please. I'm not finished."

Jillian alternated between holding her head and expressing shock at the six beers she had—"Oh, I can't believe what I've done!"—and hitting on Baby on the next stool. Jillian mentioned something about "Later on." I wondered what her professor thought of her parents.

"Where'd you get this stuff?" I asked. "I mean drinking and flirting and, you know, women in cages."

"The Disney Channel," she said.

"Oh. Okay then. Carry on."

She proceeded. It was both alarming and pleasing, like the time in grade school when she had referred to a boy in her class as a "deck." We were impressed with Jillian's imagination and ease of expression. The content though . . .

Jillian ended by leaving Baby at the bar. Thank God.

"I gotta go home," she explained, "and sleep this one off."

In the car the next morning, Jillian asked me what I thought of her performance.

"I give it a 70, Dick," I said. "Good words, but I couldn't dance to it."

Jillian said, "Da-a-a-d."

From the backseat, Ryan said, "What does that mean, sir?"

We arrived at school at the appointed hour. As was my drop-off custom, I announced, "Yet another on-time arrival from Daugherty Airlines!" Jillian rolled her eyes and informed me that the car was not an airplane. Ryan, as was his custom, chanted along with me, knowing it irritated his girlfriend. As they exited, I said, "Have a wonderful, fabulous, amazing, incredible, mesmerizing, fantastic . . ."

They'd be through the doors of the BPE Building before I ever finished. "Day," I said to myself.

CHAPTER 25

Dave Bezold

We change each other's lives.
That's the beauty of collaboration.
—KELLE LEMLEY

Dave Bezold is the men's basketball coach at NKU. He would have found Jillian Daugherty eventually. People like Bezold are meant for people like Jillian, and vice versa.

In March 2010, Bezold and I appeared on a sports talk-radio program at a restaurant just off the NKU campus. We were there to talk about the upcoming NCAA tournament. Dave had something else in mind.

"Do you think Jillian would like to be a manager for the basketball team?" he asked.

Dave didn't know Jillian, but he knew of her. He made it his business to know people who wouldn't let an errant spin of life's wheel slow them down. He'd been dealing with them his whole life. He married a woman who grew up the same way, on a farm in Wisconsin. Being gracious was inevitable.

"No guarantees," he said. "I don't want anybody feeling like this will be a sideshow. She needs to be able to operate within our family. She has to work. If it doesn't work out, we'll at least know we tried."

I posed the question to Jillian later that night. Her answer didn't require a lot of thought. A new set of homeys? Potentially an updated "home dawg" to take Evan Stanley's place? Jillian gets a trill in her voice when she's unusually excited. Her pitch is a note or two higher on the scale. "Wha-a-a-t?" she said when I told her the news. "Yes! Yes!"

I told her nothing was guaranteed. "Coach Bezold said he'll give you a shot, and see how it goes."

"Oh, it'll go great," said Jillian. "Don't you worry about that, Daddy-O."

Not long afterward, Kerry took Jillian to Bezold's office for an interview. The coach explained Jillian's duties in detail. She would fill water bottles at practice, mop the basketball floor, be in charge of passing out fresh towels to sweaty players. During games, Jillian would get water for players during timeouts and keep the towels coming. She would do whatever the head manager, Danny Boehmker, told her to do.

Bezold asked Jillian if she had any questions. Jillian said no. She could handle the job.

"I'll give you my phone number, if you think of anything," Bezold said.

Jillian took her cell phone from her purse to add the contact. "Okay," she asked, "what's your name?"

Jillian has never lived anywhere but Ohio, but she took the best from people who came from all over. It's not a stretch to say Jillian was raised in Nancy Croskey's New York and in the Chicago of Martha Cummings, in the pastoral beauty of a region in southwestern Wisconsin known as the Driftless, and in the suburbs of northern Kentucky, just across the river from Ohio.

Dave Bezold grew up in northern Kentucky, along with his four brothers, a sister, two parents and anyone needing a place to stay. A knock at the door could mean just about anything. Most often, it meant Dave would be spending the night on the couch in the living room.

"My dad believed there was good in everyone, and that people need to take care of each other" is Bezold's explanation.

Frank Bezold raised six kids in a four-bedroom house. He was a schoolteacher. For many years, he taught in parochial schools that offered neither a pension nor health insurance. The family didn't have a lot left over. The Bezolds never ran out of money before they ran out of month, though it could be a photo finish. Especially since Frank had an affinity for saving the world. Or at least his tiny piece of it, one temporarily lost soul at a time. "We took in strays," Dave explained. "It wasn't a halfway house. But it wasn't far from it sometimes."

Lots of Dave's stories start, "When I was in (fill in the school grade) a guy (or girl) came to the door with a suitcase and stayed for (days, weeks, months)." Frank's first stray, as Dave recalls, was a teacher friend who was going through a divorce. "He was living in his car," Dave says.

As Frank Bezold recalls it, the conversation went like this: "Where'd you stay last night?"

"In the White Castle parking lot."

"Okay. Come on. We're putting you up."

Dave remembers giving up his bed and spending several months after that sleeping on the living room couch. The precedent had been set.

Actually, Frank and Trudy had warmed it up a few years earlier. Exchange students from Mexico and Germany attended NKU. They arrived to find that all the campus living options had been exhausted. The Bezolds had their first boarders.

Early on, the German student was puzzled. He asked the Bezolds at dinner, "Aren't you going to put your feet up on the table?" Trudy Bezold can't recall if that was before or after the student expressed amazement that the Bezolds actually wore shoes. "He'd made some assumptions about Kentucky," she explained.

The strays arrived at a regular pace: Kids who'd left home, kids who'd been thrown out. An uncle who was building a house and needed a place to stay that had a suitable roof. The family was never quite sure who'd be at the breakfast table in the morning or on the couch at night. It could be a friend of their children who'd been over-served the night before and didn't need to be driving. It could be another kid needing to escape the negative noise of his own house.

Dave never felt burdened by the way station he called home. He never knew anything else. "We just knew that you take care of people."

It was no coincidence that in college Dave became attracted to Lisa Lemley. Her circumstances might have been different; her family narrative was fundamentally similar. In

1971, Lisa's father, Bud, decided to reinvent himself, along with the life of his family. Bud moved his wife and two daughters from a Chicago suburb to 120 rural acres in southwest Wisconsin, where people lived communally. Their lives depended on interdependence.

From a restored Victorian in Evanston, Bud led his somewhat bewildered family to a run-down four-room farmhouse without electricity or running water. Bud called the place "Shalom," Hebrew for "peace." It was in an area of Wisconsin known as the Driftless, for its lack of glacial activity. The nearest town was Viroqua, population 4,000, 20 minutes away.

Bud had been a stockbroker in Chicago; in Wisconsin, he became a farmer. Bud knew nothing about farming. He started with a one-acre plot near the farmhouse, where he planted vegetables, including two neat 60-foot rows of lettuce. This was a source of amusement for the local farmers, who knew that to feed a family of four enough lettuce for a year, a man need only plant two rows, two feet each. Bud Lemley had planted enough lettuce for a small nation of rabbits. As Lisa recalled, "People drove by and said, 'There's the idiot from Chicago.'"

Bud was not deterred. He didn't leave Chicago because he wanted to become a farmer, even though farming was what he would do. He left seeking a more cooperative, less cynical way to live. He heated the house with wood; the walls were insulated with newspapers. The family ate from wooden bowls, with wooden spoons.

"Subsistence living," said Bud's wife, Katie.

After six months, they moved to a larger piece of land that the Lemleys shared with another family. The parcel had two houses, each with indoor plumbing. "Heaven," Katie Lemley called it. The idea of fleeing the city for a "simpler" life was not unusual in 1971. "Hundreds of families did it," Katie said, including the family with whom they shared the second farm.

The two families started a dairy operation with a herd of cattle and 50 goats. Goat cheese made the families a little money, but it wasn't enough. Katie Lemley took a job as a nurse at a hospital 30 minutes away. Idealistic notions aside, Shalom was not an idyll. "I just got worn out. The simple life is not simple," Katie said. Long physical hours, for what amounted to minimum wage, took their toll.

Seven years after they'd arrived, the Lemleys kept the farm but moved back to the city. The grand experiment was over, with no regrets. The war in Vietnam had ended two years earlier, the country no longer raged within itself. Bud went back to being a broker. The lessons learned at Shalom did not fade though.

"It's easy to live well with your neighbor when nobody has anything," Katie Lemley said. "Everybody lived the same. We shared everything."

Or as Kelle Lemley, Lisa's sister, put it, "We helped each other. Helping each other was the only way we survived."

The Driftless has become a booming region for the organic-food movement that started in the late 1960s with families like the Lemleys. The spirit of giving and receiving gracefully lives on. Communal farms are common. So too are formerly suburban families, looking for a different way to be.

Bud and Katie have moved back to the farm permanently. Bud runs his own brokerage now, from an outbuilding on their property. Whenever Bud has money, he gives a lot of it away.

He isn't specific, nor are his family members, about where the money goes. "When I've had money, I've shared it. I've put some kids through college" is all he says.

Kelle is an assistant professor in the College of Education at Northern Arizona University, where she remains active in social causes. Lisa married Dave Bezold. Their past lives inform their current lifestyle.

Dave's grandparents, his father Frank's parents, took in two of his elderly aunts when they could no longer live on their own. Dave's mother, Trudy, was one of eleven children. There were no assisted-living places then, and even if there were, nobody had the money to pay for them. Taking care of one another didn't come with angel's wings. "People helped us. We helped them. It's just what you did," Trudy said.

The people fit no mold. Or as Dave puts it, "So you have six earrings in your nose and your hair is blue, we don't care about that. It took us out of our comfort zone. We were taught to keep our eyes open. There's something good about everybody. There are no strangers out there."

Sometimes now, when the NKU basketball team is on an extended road trip and Lisa isn't at home, Frank will go to his son's house to bring in the mail and the newspapers and to see if everything is normal. He'll walk in and be greeted by people, students usually, whom he's never seen. He'll chuckle then and be proud of how he raised his son.

Jillian arrived at basketball practice on October 15, 2010, and nearly every day thereafter, for three years. The only expectation Dave had of her was that she do her best and make a contribution. Jillian's only requirement was that she be accepted and respected as part of the team.

We're only as good as the way we treat each other. Kindness is a cumulative act. It builds.

"Jillian makes me laugh every day," Bezold said not long ago. "She makes me think every day. She makes me happy every day. I wish I had that in me."

As with every meaningful transaction involving Jillian and the world, each side profited. Jillian got the belonging of the basketball team, and the validation taken from being a functioning part of a typical work setting. Dave Bezold didn't give Jillian a sense of place. He gave her the place itself. The whole room.

The basketball team got the Jillian Daugherty Show, guileless and mirthful, every last syllable and chorus. Their coach rediscovered how to laugh in a pure way, free of complication, the way young children do. The players discovered that different is good.

The Bezolds and the Lemleys chose to take part in the human community. Their villages became Jillian's. All those strays and neighbors and kids needing money for college were better for having known them. No better, though, than their benefactors, who learned that receiving is the happy and often unintended consequence of giving.

Jillian keeps the circle unbroken. She validates Shalom. Bud Lemley's lettuce kingdom lives on, paid forward, in the life of a young lady he has never met.

"I love my team," Jillian says every once in a while, just because.

CHAPTER 26

The Team

Today is here. Let's not waste it.
—DANNY BOEHMKER, NKU
BASKETBALL MANAGER

Jillian could negotiate the bus lines. She'd gotten to know the campus well enough that she'd begun helping with tours for prospective students with disabilities. Jillian was comfortable spending the entire day at NKU. All she needed was an outlet for her considerable social ambitions—a broader audience for the Jillian Daugherty Show

The basketball experiment that began in Jillian's second year sprang from Dave Bezold's heart and evolved through Jillian's personality. It needed more than that. As with all of Jillian's social endeavors, it required a broader acceptance. Bezold could declare that Jillian would be a manager for his team. He could inform all involved, as he did, some individually. But Bezold couldn't make his players accept Jillian, or respect her, or even be comfortable in her presence. The Jillian Show was lonely without co-stars.

The welcoming had to start somewhere other than by decree of the head coach. It started with Danny Boehmker. Boehmker grew up with an uncle who had Down syndrome. Uncle Denny was Danny's father's brother, the last of four sons of parents who ran a bar in Covington, Kentucky, across the Ohio River from Cincinnati. Denny Boehmker's disability was severe, and the era in which he grew up was not sympathetic. Denny never spoke.

As an adult, he split his days between a menial job and his favorite chair at Herb and Thelma's bar, greeting patrons whether he knew them or not. If a newcomer sat in Denny's chair, it wasn't for long. His pleasures were as limited as his world. Denny watched TV and listened to music. He enjoyed playing with a balloon attached to the end of a string. He died on Christmas Day nine years ago, at age 46, never having said a word.

Communication isn't just language, though. And dying is just a physical act. Denny endured in the memories and deeds of those who knew him best. "He brought love to our family," said Danny's father, Chip. "He kept us together."

Danny spent a lot of time with his uncle. There was something about Denny that he couldn't let go. A feeling, he says. They communicated in a way that both understood. They'd roll a ball back and forth between them. Danny would yank on the string tied to the balloon. Denny would laugh. He had an easy laugh.

So when Dave Bezold named Danny head manager and informed him that Jillian Daugherty would be his assistant, Danny felt blessed. The way he saw it, he'd teach Jillian how to fold towels and keep water bottles filled. Jillian would further his education on how to be a good human being.

That's how Bezold saw it too: "She gets a chance to grow and be part of something. Jillian needs that. That's part of her personality. She loves an audience. My guys get to experience someone who is different from them."

There's something good about everybody. There are no strangers out there.

The players didn't accept Jillian right away. They looked at someone who didn't look like them, whose words they didn't always understand and whose disability they'd never experienced, certainly not on a daily basis. They were hesitant, even fearful. It would take time. With Jillian, it always takes time. But for her, the ritual belonging never fades. She is the most people of persons. For Jillian, being "one of the guys" is not an expression. It is a central happiness of her life. The basketball partnership would fortify that happiness yet again.

"Do you want to learn to Dougie?" Danny asked her.

This question came after she'd been on the job a few weeks, feeling her way. At first, Jillian's biggest job was to be at practice on time and to follow Danny around. She could do that. She was also being uncharacteristically shy. "Coach Beez" did not have time during practice to worry about his newest manager. Jillian wasn't "special" to him. She was the rookie manager, and she'd better have the water bottles filled and the sweat wiped from the practice floor.

Jillian did not immediately take to the new routine. She

was intimidated and overwhelmed, two new emotions for her. "At first, she was afraid to show any feelings at all," Danny recalled. "She'd walk away, behind the bleachers, if she was mad or sad. She was hesitant to ask questions. The players initially didn't know what to do with her."

But Jillian could dance. She could always dance.

"I want to do the Dougie," Jillian said to Danny.

He showed her the basics. The Dougie is a hip-hop creation named for the rapper Doug E. Fresh. It was first performed in 2007 or so. To the untrained eye—that is, the old-guy eye like mine who knew the Twist and the Jerk, oh so many seasons ago—the Dougie is a modified shimmy-shoulder roll during which you pass your hands by the sides of your head. There is no right or wrong way to Dougie, which made it perfect for Jillian.

For the next week, when Danny arrived at practice, Jillian was already there, working on her Dougie. She'd be standing at center court with her headphones on, alone in the gym, shoulder-shimmying, running her hands past the sides of her head. She did it at home, too, in the basement, in front of the mirror, the same as she did when she was practicing for her high school dance team.

She broke it out before practice one day about a month into her managing career. Some players laughed with her; some laughed at her. Jillian thought it was all good. That's the thing about her particular disability and her personality: Jillian always assumes laughter to be positive.

She understands outright meanness. Derisive laughter is more subtle. It's harder for her to process. Jillian thought the players were in total acceptance mode. Danny knew this wasn't the case and would talk individually to those who had gotten a kick out of his co-worker for the wrong reasons.

Jillian was undeterred. In fact, she was emboldened. The way she saw it, these new home-dogs were welcoming her. They liked her Dougie.

From there, it was only a small leap of audacity for Jillian to assume the entire team would enjoy her talents as a rapper. Jillian was an enthusiastic rapper, honing her skills with Eminem and Snoop Dogg CDs she'd liberated from her brother. To put it politely, Jillian wasn't especially polished with rhymes. Imagine Tupac doing Shakespeare at the Globe. At first, she practiced only in front of Danny. If she came up with a new rap at home, she'd call Danny. Sometimes, if Danny was with his family or girlfriend, he'd put Jillian on speakerphone so everyone could enjoy her rhymes. Jillian made Danny laugh, every time.

By January, Jillian apparently felt ready for the footlights. I say apparently because Kerry and I had no idea she'd been plotting her rapping debut until long after it happened. That was probably for the best because if we'd gotten wind of it, we might have stopped it. That's probably why Jillian never gave us a clue.

She asked Coach Beez if she could rap for the team. Fortunately, Beez didn't ask for a sample. If he had, Jillian would never have desecrated a rhyme in public. Instead, Bezold said, "Okay, but it better be good."

"Oh, it will be," Jillian said.

On the day of her first public rapping appearance, which would occur immediately after practice, Jillian spent most of practice in a luxury box on the second level of the Bank of Kentucky Center, the 9,400-seat arena on the NKU campus. Players heard strange sounds coming from the box and wondered whose cat was being tortured. At the end of practice, at a time Bezold had approved in advance, Jillian yelled, "Yo!Yo!Yo! Listen up, y'all!"

The players looked up to see their new manager as she edged from the luxury box. Jillian's basketball shorts rode low on her hips. She wore her ball cap sideways. She danced— the Dougie, perhaps—as she rolled down a very long flight of steps.

"Give it up for J-Dog!" she said.

What?

The players were amused—and some of them were snickering at her. Undeterred, Jillian busted a few Snoop-inspired rhymes. When she was done, the players applauded, sort of.

After that first excursion, there was no stopping her, and as the days and weeks rolled by, the players bought into this version of the Jillian Daugherty Show. They saw Jillian come to practice every day. They saw her fill their water bottles and keep their court dry as they practiced. They saw her passion during games. They felt her encouragement, no matter how well they played. They started to realize her support for them was unconditional and her work ethic was genuine. Jillian's aim was true.

Soon enough, she had worked out an arrangement with Coach Beez. Each Friday after practice, she would get 35 seconds—a full shot clock—to address the team with a rap. When the buzzer sounded, she'd have to stop lest the rap session last all weekend.

Jillian became expert at mentioning individual players. She

knew their birthdays. She picked up on their unique traits, usually by listening to Bezold during practice. Tony Rack, for example, was a very good three-point shooter. Thus:

"There goes Tony, my three-point homey."

She noticed the coaching staff's practice exhortations: Box out. Stay tight. Rebound. If Bezold had gotten on a particular player during practice, she'd work that into the rhyme:

"Coach Beez mad, Malcolm sad. But it gonna be all right, yeah!"

Players were especially amused by those rhymes. Jocks aren't sparing with the mutual ridicule. Jillian also knew who NKU's next opponent was and would trash-talk that team. Soon the players dubbed Jillian's shows Freestyle Friday. She'd begin working on that week's rhymes a day in advance, then call Danny on Thursday nights to test them out. Poor Danny. He heard more bad tunes than the judges on *American Idol*.

The quality wasn't important, of course. Jillian rapped with utter authenticity and transparency. She had no agenda beyond wanting to be one of the guys. The guys saw that, and the players who'd been uncomfortable initially with Jillian started asking her to feature them in that week's rap.

By the time Jillian was a third-year manager, her rapping had become a highlight of Friday practices. The rhymes didn't define Jillian's role with the team though. They were her entry, but they didn't allow for the whole Jillian Daugherty Show.

That first year, she became enamored with Tony Rack. He was a junior guard with a surpassing work ethic and desire to win. He was a crazy man. We say this in the nicest of ways. Jillian leaned on Danny Boehmker, but she worshipped Tony. Her relationship with all "my players," as she called them, was important. Her affection for Rack was something more.

"I love my man Tony," she'd say. After her first game as a manager, Jillian brought Tony over to meet us. "This is Tony Rack," she said. "He's my best man."

Rack was a local guy, raised in the Cincinnati suburbs. He had attended Moeller High School, just across the river in Montgomery, Ohio. He'd never known anyone with a disability, let alone someone like Jillian. It was an uneasy pairing at first. Jillian made a point of buying her new best man snacks and drinks, which she'd present to him before almost every practice. It made Rack uneasy to the point where he asked Danny and Bezold to talk to Jillian about it.

"I didn't know how to handle it," Rack recalled years later. "I didn't want to hurt her, but I didn't want to take her money."

Early on, Rack was the only player Jillian talked to. This embarrassed Tony who, despite his outgoing nature, was uncomfortable with the attention. Things changed eventually, as Jillian loosened up and other players became comfortable with her. But Jillian's fondness for Tony never wavered, and she showed that by joking with him.

One game his junior year, Rack had just come off the floor after badly missing a three-pointer. It was late in a game NKU had well in hand. Jillian fulfilled her duties by fetching Tony a towel and a cup of water. But not without a dig:

"The way you're shooting tonight," she said, "you're lucky I don't pour this on you."

Also in his junior season, Rack drilled a three-pointer at the buzzer to beat Kentucky Wesleyan in an NCAA Tournament game. It was among the biggest shots of his career. Just before the shot, during a timeout, Bezold walked to the far end of the bench where Jillian stood guard over the watercooler.

"You're going to draw up a play for Tony to take the last shot, right?" she asked the coach.

But it was during the bad times that Jillian was most instructive. Rack injured his shoulder as a senior. The pain was so intense he took a cortisone injection to numb it, and eventually even that didn't help. On Senior Night, the pain was such that Rack cried during warm-ups. He started the game, then took himself out 30 seconds into it. "The only time I'd ever done that," he recalled.

He never left the bench after that, and NKU lost the game. Rack was inconsolable afterward. He didn't feel much like talking, to anyone. As he walked down the hallway from the court to the locker room, Rack felt a basketball thump him in the rear.

What the . . . ? He wasn't in the mood. He turned around quickly. This could be a problem.

"You're still my home dawg, Tony Rack," Jillian said. "Even if you're hurt, I still got your back."

JILLIAN TOOK LOSSES HARD too. A few times in her first season, Kerry and I had to counsel her not to let her emotions flow during the game. "You have a job to do. You can't be getting upset," we'd say.

But the disappointment never lasted with her. Once the game was over, it was over. "With her, it's in the moment," Rack said. "That's the way it should be."

Jillian would get very concerned about how the players felt. That's why she tossed the ball at Rack. It was why, before every road game, Jillian figured when the team would be on the bus, from the hotel to the gym, and called Danny's cell phone.

Jillian didn't go with them for the roadies because everyone had a roommate, and she was the only female. That disappointed her more than anything. Still, she guessed the team needed her so she lent her support long distance, either with a pep talk or a rap. Danny put her on speakerphone. The bus got quiet whenever she called. On the rare occasions Jillian missed the timing for the call, players would wonder what happened. A few times, Danny called her from the back of the bus.

Not long ago, I asked Tony Rack what Jillian had taught him. They were together two years. Not a day passed when Jillian didn't talk about her best man. Eventually, the feeling became mutual. "She gave me the realization that everyone is a role model," Rack said. "No matter what I was doing, someone was watching. Like that cussing after I missed a shot.

"People always watched her, too," partly, Rack allowed candidly, because of her disability. "She was always doing her best, on her best behavior. I think she felt the eyes on her."

Kevin Schappell is an assistant coach. He attended Loveland High, where he was a local star, before Jillian got there. But he knew about her by the time she got to NKU. Assistants do the bulk of the recruiting of high school players. Teams that don't recruit well don't win, no matter the competence of their coaches.

"Any connection you can make with a recruit and his family helps," Schappell said.

One year, the mother of NKU's most coveted recruit had a nephew with Down syndrome. Schappell got Jillian to help with the recruiting process. The family met her, and she talked about her job, her classes and the life she had on campus. "The mother broke down in tears," Schappell said. And the player signed with Northern Kentucky.

Kindness builds. Respect is established. Jillian becomes part of the team, and the human transaction Bezold hoped would happen did occur.

"Open your eyes and you will see the good in everybody," Bezold said. "Jillian shows my players that everyone has something to contribute. They need to know the importance of taking care of people. I can tell them that. But I'm a 45-year-old guy. For them to experience it is irreplaceable. That's what college is, a place to give these kids as many experiences as possible. That's how they grow. We have all kinds of kids here. Country kids, inner-city kids. Kids who've never seen anyone that doesn't look like them. They need that exposure. Basketball is basketball."

Jillian gave the players another prism through which to see the world. Her optimism and agenda-free friendship let them know that while basketball was temporary, how they chose to live their lives was indelible.

Jillian's duties expanded with her confidence. She went from filling water bottles and folding towels to washing practice uniforms. She learned the codes to all the locker-room doors. During practice, she'd slip over her arms what looked like a big foam shield. As players dribbled, she'd whack them with the shield to simulate a persistent defender, albeit one that was a full two feet shorter than they were.

"Box out!" she'd yell, sometimes too zealously. Bezold would rein that in on occasion, especially if the team was practicing fast breaks. "Stay tight!" "Rebound!"

On most school days, Jillian was in Bezold's office by noon, after her classes had concluded, studying or reading on his couch, waiting for practice to start. She'd have a Ryan story, or a tale of something that had happened at home. Dave Bezold knew more about our family than we did.

As the players grew to enjoy her, they embraced and protected her. They sang "Happy Birthday" to her. She invited them to a summer picnic at our house. Several made it. A year after Rack graduated, he called her to wish her happy birthday. Upperclassmen would break in the newcomers: "That's J-Dawg. Treat her with respect."

"She never fails to do something enjoyable," Boehmker decided. I'd asked him too, what does Jillian teach?

"Just to slow down sometimes," Danny said. "She's a reminder that today is here. Let's not waste it."

We meet in our lives any number of people who profess to love us and care about us. Some might actually mean it. With Jillian, there's never a doubt. The players knew that. Eventually. All of them.

Jillian validated Bezold's belief in helping others to the betterment of ourselves. If you love someone, Jillian said, they'll love you back.

A few weeks after Tony Rack's final game at Northern Kentucky, I got an e-mail from his parents:

> When NKU lost its basketball game in the NCAA tournament, it brought an end to their season. It was also the end of our son Tony's basketball career. A career that lasted 14 years.
>
> After the loss, our family and friends were sitting in

the empty bleachers with Tony. It was a very emotional time for all of us. Then a small little angel came walking across the gym floor. It was your Jillian.

She told him she enjoyed being on the team with him and she was glad they became good friends. Jillian turned to me and said, "Don't be sad about today, be proud of the way Tony Rack played. He always tried his best."

She turned back to Tony and said "Tony Rack, I am going to miss you." Tony was still sitting in the bleachers and looked almost level to her and said, "Jillian, I am going to miss you a lot, too. You worked as hard as anyone on this team. Your encouragement inspired me in ways you will never know."

Jillian said, "Tony, our bus is waiting to take the team back to NKU. Are you ready?" He looked over at us and said, "I am now. Let's get on the bus together."

I cannot tell you how much her words meant to us. Sometimes God sends a little angel to get you through the hard times. I cannot even remember the score of that last game, but I will never forget Jillian's kindness.

Back at the arena, Jillian is tossing dirty practice uniforms into an industrial-size washing machine. "I can't wait for Friday," she says to Danny. "It's going to be my best rap ever."

Danny smiles, knowing what he knows. Today is here. Let's not waste it. "I'm sure it will be, J-Dog," he says.

CHAPTER 27

Jillian Turns 21

*A love that takes us out of ourselves and binds us to
something larger. We know that's what matters.*
—PRESIDENT BARACK OBAMA, AT A MEMORIAL
SERVICE FOR THE FAMILIES OF THE SLAIN
CHILDREN OF NEWTOWN, CONNECTICUT

Jillian celebrated the rest of us all the time. Every so often,
the rest of us celebrated Jillian. She turned 21 on a Sunday in
October. We let people know we were going to note the milestone by gathering at a local sports bar, where well-wishers
could watch the guest of honor drink her first beer, an event
she'd anticipated for months.

"I can't wait until I get my first beer," Jillian would announce
at random moments. That made for interesting conversation
with her teachers, friends and parents of friends. Jillian was not
deterred.

It was to be an informal affair. Beer, appetizers, football on the big screens. Come when you will, go when you like. We figured 20 to 30 people would be there: Kelly, his girlfriend, Ruby, both sets of grandparents, longtime family friends, people from the neighborhood. The restaurant pulled together two eight-top tables and assigned us one server for the four hours we intended to stay.

Close to 70 people showed up.

Friends, family, neighbors. People we didn't know and had never seen. They just dropped by. "All these people are here because of you," I said to Jillian, a few hours into it.

"I don't know what to say, Dad," she said. "I love my life."

I tried to summon some significance beyond the obvious. I looked for the water pressure behind the eyes. Jillian was 21 years old and thriving. An outward display of emotion seemed the way to go. It didn't happen. Twenty-one was like graduation, like Jillian's first day at Northern Kentucky.

The pride we felt on Jillian's major days was the same we felt with Kelly's. We'd planned for them, we'd worked for them. We'd expected them. Jillian did the rest. When they occurred, we noted them and celebrated them. At that point, tears would have been something of a conceit: Look what we've done for our 21-year-old with a disability.

The smaller moments elicited tears though. The little wins prompted them.

"I'm a big girl now," Jillian had said that morning on her birthday.

"You've been a big girl for a while," I said.

"Now I'm official," Jillian said. And then this:

"Dad, I'm so happy now. I'm your little girl, and I get to drink beer. Thank you and Mom for being the best parents to me. You guys are the best. I know I'm going to move out soon, and I will miss you guys. But I will always love you."

"Thank you, Jills. You're moving out?"

"Well, not right away, Dad. But soon. I know you'll be a wreck."

"Probably," I said. "And Jillian?"

"Yeah?"

"One beer today."

My mother and father sat quietly in the back, away from the thick of the festivities, which were centered around Jillian's high-top table. They'd come from Florida for the party. They'd moved to the gulf coast in 1982, when my dad was 49 years old. He'd worked for the federal government for 25 years. He'd had enough. My mother's parents had retired in Bradenton, and she wanted to be close to them.

I was 24 years old when they moved; my brother and sister were 27. Eventually, my sister moved to the same town, but my brother and I stayed north, he in Maryland, I in Ohio. A family, separated by a thousand miles. Absentee love. The distance created a regret my mother has only recently expressed. Five grandchildren have grown up seeing their grandparents only for a few days in the summertime and on the occasional Christmas visit. Love was given and received on the telephone, in thank-you notes, in well wishes after graduations and traditional holidays. It was abiding but fleeting.

More than 30 years after my parents moved to Florida, they wish they hadn't. At least not so soon. Being closer to one part of the family meant more distance from the rest of us. My mother never got to know her grandchildren. "I missed out on all of it," she said.

She and my dad had planned to stay an hour or two at the party, then retreat back to our house. They aren't big on socializing and are less enthusiastic about large crowds. Instead, they stayed the entire time. My father, whose affinity for grandparenting was tepid at best, was genuinely moved by the occasion.

"Write about this," he said. "People need to know how this works."

How this works. What an apt phrase.

Jillian embraced all her family, even the members who weren't related to her. Sometimes, especially those people. Dave Bezold and Danny Boehmker. Evan Stanley and Tony Rack. These weren't simply friends to Jillian. They were essential relationships, as defining and meaningful as any she had.

Jillian had the basic support of a nuclear clan. Most of us have that, whether out of love or obligation or both. Jillian inspired a larger family.

These were people who, from a distance, made her life better. They came together on days such as this one, not out of obligation (they had none) or love (not in the literal, family sense), but because they knew she genuinely appreciated their presence. And because wishing Jillian well made them feel better about themselves.

This was how it worked.

Kerry's parents, Sid and Jean, were part of the Jillian posse. They lived close enough—in Pittsburgh, not quite five hours away—to come for birthdays and Christmas and special moments in between. My parents loved from a distance. On this day, they realized a little of what that distance had caused them to miss—especially because I wasn't great at getting my kids down to Florida on even a semi-regular basis.

Jillian would always have a strong, blood-related family. We were her base camp, from which further exploration was possible. The legions of other family members allowed her to roam. They broadened the confidence we instilled. Without them, Jillian would not be Jillian.

Her 21st birthday would go on for a week. Every day, someone would give her a present or take her to lunch. The basketball team sang "Happy Birthday" to her. An assistant coach baked cupcakes for her. In the middle of the seemingly endless tributes, I asked her, "Do you know why people are always so nice to you?"

We were in the car, on the way to NKU, where the women's basketball coaching staff was taking Jillian to lunch that day.

"Because I'm a good person?" Jillian answered.

Yes.

Back at the sports bar, a man named Bob Young said, "Thanks for inviting me." I'd met Bob once before. He's a regular contributor to the blog I write for the *Enquirer*. He'd never met Jillian. He'd read about the party and had brought along his college-age son. "What an inspiration Jillian is," he said.

The inspiration worked the crowd. "Thank you for coming to my party," Jillian said. "Nice to meet you. Are you having a good time?" People were attracted to her. People she'd never met. A wonder of Jillian is the joy she inspires in others. Her disability enables.

They came and went on a fine autumn Sunday, when they

could have been doing something else. We thanked them all. I wanted to ask them why they came. But I knew. I knew why they came.

Jillian ordered a Sam Adams Light at 1:00 p.m., as soon as we arrived. At 5:00 p.m., she finished it. "I loved my beer, Dad," she said as we walked from the restaurant. "I loved my day."

CHAPTER 28

Testing

They're grieving for the loss of perfect.
—DR. RONALD JAEKLE, DIRECTOR OF
PERINATAL SERVICES, UNIVERSITY
OF CINCINNATI HOSPITAL

Modern science has made it possible to grieve and celebrate all at once. In some corners, science is capable of pounding both sides of the same drum, producing sounds so different, you wouldn't dream they'd be coming from the same instrument.

Just as Jillian Daugherty and her big family gathered to celebrate her present and future, doctors and researchers were working to make it meaningless. You don't have to have a child with Down syndrome now. An expectant mother can undergo something called nuchal translucency screening. It's as easy as a finger prick and a blood draw, and it's done between the 11th and 14th weeks of pregnancy. Even then, fetal

DNA floats freely in the mother's bloodstream. Technically, the test doesn't provide a diagnosis of Down syndrome; it tells a woman if she is at increased risk. But the test does identify between 85 and 95 percent of Down syndrome babies, which makes it a rather accurate forecast.

"Prenatal technology," they call it. Building better babies through medical breakthroughs. Bioengineering is not science fiction. It's science.

What would you do?

It's rare now that hospitals suggest that parents of a new-born with Down syndrome give the baby up for adoption. It's all but unheard of that parents are asked if they intend to keep their child. Instead, the option is entirely preemptive. Don't have the child at all.

Nuchal translucency screening was not available in 1989; amniocentesis was. Kerry's could not be performed. We had no decision to make, a non-occurrence for which I still say prayers.

It's easier than ever to make everything right. Bodies are worked like pieces of clay. Tightened and tucked. Parts are replaced, lines are erased. Parents start preparing their kinder-garten kids for college. Heaven help them if they're not playing Select soccer or Beethoven by the age of ten.

None of us is perfect. Some of us try to be. Others see it as a right.

A forecast of a child with a "chromosomal abnormality" doesn't meet anyone's definition of perfect. Today about 90 percent of women who are told they're likely to have a baby born with Down syndrome will choose to abort. That is the cold, hard calculus in the age of designer children.

Science doesn't get a free pass, though. It squirms in the presence of moral judgment. Are we making choices that aren't ours to make? Do we have the right to have a "perfect" child? If we do, define perfection. Is it permissible to wipe out an entire segment of the population? What becomes of those left in that group, when humans like them can be so easily eliminated?

"So many people are focused on the negative aspect," says Dr. Ronald Jaekle. He is a professor of clinical ob-gyn at the University of Cincinnati Medical School. He's also the director of perinatal services at University Hospital there. "None of us were guaranteed a perfect life."

Dr. Jaekle does between 30 and 35 ultrasounds a day. One in 25 will reveal a birth defect. He welcomes the nuchal screening. Not for the life-or-death option it provides, but for the preparedness it offers. Prepared parents are better parents, he says. "Parents with the pre-natal diagnosis are more effective parents for the first two or three years of the child's life," he says. "That's our only goal here."

Dr. Jaekle disputes the high termination rate. He claims that "less than 5 percent" of his patients choose to terminate the pregnancy. "I get frustrated when someone's baby has a non-lethal anomaly, and they wonder if they should terminate. It's not my place to make that decision. I'll explain the reasons they shouldn't, but I'm not going to be judgmental."

At that point, the doctor functions as an unofficial grief counselor.

"That's their biggest reaction. They think they're grieving for the loss of the baby. They're really grieving for the loss of perfect. Women during a pregnancy sculpt their kids' entire lives. What color dress for senior prom? What about the wedding? It's a storybook. That's where the grief comes in. It's a normal response we want to work through."

Mothers aren't the only ones lost in that dream. Before Jillian was born, I imagined cymbidium orchids under a porch light.

Dr. Jaekle doesn't come to the subject blindly. His 25-year-old daughter Melissa was born 13 weeks premature with cerebral palsy. She weighed 2 pounds, 13 ounces. Five minutes after her birth, Melissa was still receiving chest compressions and had an Apgar score of zero. "You don't have to do this for us," Dr. Jaekle told the medical staff keeping his baby girl alive.

Melissa survived. She spent the first year of her life in the hospital. Doctors told the Jaekles their daughter likely wouldn't walk or talk. Melissa has thrived, thanks to informed and insistent parents. "The biggest challenge has always been making sure everyone else had the same expectations for Melissa that we did," said Dr. Jaekle.

Armed with that vast continent of empathy, the doctor addresses couples at one of the biggest crossroads of their lives.

"My job is to get them to come to terms with what we have found," Dr. Jaekle said. "What we traditionally say is, 'You need to recognize that the overwhelming majority of the kids with Down syndrome are valued and valuable members of their family.' It's not a devastating end, just a different direction. I want them to be able to embrace this different future and go forward."

Tough sell, that.

On the surface, the answer couldn't be easier. Do you want a child with a disability, or a child without one?

The fear doesn't end when the child is born, regardless of the preparedness. Media reports are sprinkled with parental misgivings. In a November 2011 story in *Time* magazine, a woman pregnant with a child with Down syndrome wondered what the child "would do to her marriage and her two older children."

Another story in *Time,* in February 2012, featured a new mother who admitted she waited eight hours before she "mustered the nerve" to visit her new baby girl in the neonatal intensive care unit. "I was so afraid of what she was going to look like," she said.

Even Ron Jaekle said it took him "many years" to come to terms with Melissa's disability.

It doesn't help that society can still view people with cognitive disabilities as lesser beings, an image the media sometimes does not discourage. In 2012, political commentator Ann Coulter referred to President Obama as a "retard." Baltimore Ravens quarterback Joe Flacco used the Super Bowl stage in February 2013 to label "retarded" the notion of playing the game in a cold-weather city.

George Clooney made reference to a "retarded" individual in *The Descendants,* a movie that was nominated for an Oscar. In a November 2008 edition of the London Sunday *Times,* respected columnist Minette Marrin had this to say, in a column tangentially about abortion: "What more powerful social reason could there be for an abortion than the virtual certainty that the fetus would be condemned to a life of frustration, disappointment, dependence, serious illness and poverty, to the great sorrow and hardship of its family?"

In her biography on her website, Marrin says she has "a

special interest in learning disabilities" because "someone close to me in our family" is learning disabled. This intimate knowledge fortifies her conviction; she's the anti–Ron Jaekle.

"I am convinced that it is a grave misfortune for babies to be born with Down's or any comparably serious syndrome," Marrin writes. "It's a misfortune for their parents and their siblings as well."

Words color perception. Perception is reality. Imagine dropping the "N-word" so causally these days. We make allowances for the physical disabilities. Those with mental disabilities aren't as lucky—especially in how they are perceived.

The issue comes with the ultimate irony. Science is operating at cross-purposes when it comes to what to do with people with disabilities. Just as advanced testing threatens/promises to eliminate a whole group of people, other medical advances offer the hope that those people could thrive far beyond current expectations.

In July 2011, a story appeared in the *New York Times* about the work of Dr. Albert Costa, a physician and neuroscientist. Costa's daughter, born in 1995, has Down syndrome. Costa experimented on mice with a drug known as memantine, used to treat Alzheimer's. The results were hopeful. The mice showed improved memory. Costa concluded that they were able to learn as well as standard mice. He suggested that a similar treatment might be effective for people with cognitive disabilities.

Later that year, the Swiss biotech giant Roche announced a clinical trial "to investigate the safety and tolerability of a molecule designed to address the cognitive and behavioral deficits associated with Down syndrome." Even this research is viewed with an arched brow. Some parents of children with Down fear any improvement in intellect would come with a change in personality. They wonder if the tradeoff would be worth it.

And so it goes. There is no right or wrong answer. There is only personal experience.

Sarah Klein is Jillian's best friend. Her mother, Catherine, gave birth to Sarah, knowing Sarah would have Down syndrome. Catherine was 38 years old in 1993 so she underwent what at the time were standard tests for birth defects. Hospital staff administered an alpha-fetoprotein test, a blood draw that can detect chromosomal abnormalities in the fetus.

That result came back borderline. That day, Catherine underwent a sonogram, which showed nothing unusual, then an amniocentesis. She and her husband, Walt, were not prepared for what happened next. The phone call came days later, from her obstetrician. Walt was at work in New York City, an hour by train from their Connecticut home. Catherine had Sarah's older sister Jenny, then 18 months, in her arms when the phone rang. "You're going to have a baby girl with Down syndrome," the doctor said, with all the warmth of an audit.

"At that moment, my support group was Jenny," Catherine recalls.

The Kleins next visited a geneticist, who was equally dispassionate. He greeted them with "a litany of all that could go wrong," says Walt. "It was like an anvil falling on you." As Catherine sobbed, the doctor dispatched an intern to find some tissues. "He mentioned institutions," says Walt. "They still had them in Connecticut."

The hospital assigned the Kleins a social worker, whom

they met with three times. On each occasion, the social worker asked Catherine if she was sure she did not want to terminate the pregnancy. "It's not too late," the woman suggested.

"There seemed to be a big assumption within the medical community that I should terminate," Catherine says. She had suffered three miscarriages in a previous marriage. She never considered not having Sarah.

Walt says the couple never discussed abortion. "We were deeply in love. We mourned, but that passed quickly. We were a great family for this child. We had a great nucleus and a supportive extended family. It quickly felt like the right thing to do."

What will happen to research designed to help those with Down syndrome? The medical field might be merciful, miraculous even. It is not charitable. If the market shrinks, so will the profit motive. Just as society is grasping the benefits of including its citizens with Down syndrome, science has discovered how to eliminate them. "Weed them out" as the author of the *Time* story put it.

It's like taking one too many steps to reach the mountaintop.

Jillian wouldn't be Jillian without the enhanced and enlightened public support she has received. She would be the victim of "breakthroughs."

In the *New York Times* story, Dr. Costa says the emergence of safer and more effective prenatal testing has meant fewer dollars for Down syndrome research: Money from the National Institutes of Health plunged from $23 million in 2003 to $16 million in 2007, before rebounding to $22 million in 2011. In comparison, cystic fibrosis research received $68 million in 2011.

"If we're not quick enough to offer alternatives, this field might collapse," Costa said.

Then what?

Experience, no matter how fulfilling, is no match for scientific certainty. Condemning those who choose to abort imperfection isn't something I'm comfortable doing. I didn't walk that mile. I've walked only mine. It's been a good walk.

I don't dwell on Jillian's shortcomings any more than I do Kelly's. Neither of them is ever going to design a rocket or cure a disease, and I can live with that. Could I live without them? I'd rather not. They're good people.

I asked Walt and Catherine Klein what they might say to a couple faced with the choice the Kleins made. Sarah is 21 years old now. She graduated from high school. She's in her third year at Northern Kentucky University.

"Don't be scared" is what Catherine would say. "This child will need some extra help. Every child you have needs your help, in different ways. You can't control how your children will need you.

"A wonderful community has opened up to our entire family. The connections we've made are remarkable. Sarah has touched more lives than I will, if I live to 150."

"Come see our daughter," says Walt. "I think you'll be impressed."

Dr. Ronald Jaekle's daughter Melissa lives independently in a community for disabled adults outside Houston. "Having Melissa as a daughter has broadened my scope and allowed me to be more empathic in doing my job," Dr. Jaekle says. "It allows me to talk about the challenges, with heartfelt conviction."

Jillian Daugherty is thriving in the social mainstream, engaging and engaged, helped by a million hands, seen and unseen. The tapestry of Jillian's experience could be lost forever in the name of perfection. Which is ironic. Because in some very tangible way, Jillian is closer to perfect than anyone I've known.

CHAPTER 29

In Love and Moving Out

*I love you so much in my heart and this is amazing
we are dating for seven years. I think I want you forever. Can I keep you for my love?*
—JILLIAN, TO RYAN

On the way home from a date on a night in May 2012, the happy couple sat in the backseat of Kerry's car and dreamed aloud. The subject was their impending independence. Jillian was 22 years old, and Ryan was 24. They were ready, they decided, for their own place. They had big plans.

"We can go to Reds games," Jillian suggested, "and plant flowers."

"We can eat out whenever we want," said Ryan.

Both agreed that staying up all hours of the night would be a big plus to living together alone. There was also a mutual understanding that a dog would be involved. "I'll make you pancakes on Saturdays," Jillian suggested, "after we sleep really late."

Ryan said, "Ooooh, yeah."

Kerry and I chuckled. "Living together is a non-stop party," I said.

"We can't wait," Jillian said.

Ryan, somewhat more practical, asked, "What do you mean?"

Later that night, Jillian, Kerry and I gathered on the deck. Although Jillian enjoyed talking about leaving, and the promise of unlimited late nights and pancake breakfasts, she also had her reservations. "I'm just a little bit nervous, a little bit," she said.

"I know, Jills."

"It's going to be hard to say goodbye to you guys."

We assured her that any apartment they chose would be very close to us. We also reminded her that we didn't see her much now anyway, with her spending all day at school, managing the basketball team and the still-obligatory Jillian Daugherty Show time, in the basement or her room.

"It's true you won't be right down the hall anymore," I said. "You won't be able to tell us goodnight or give Lucy a hug." Lucy is our eight-year-old golden retriever. I wasn't trying to make Jillian feel awful, even though that's what I did. I wanted her to know that getting a place of her own wasn't all ball-games and flower boxes. "This would be a lot of hard work for you and Ryan," I said.

Jillian sniffled and pondered that for a moment. "No matter what, we stick together because we love each other," she said.

"I know you and Ryan love each other. You just need to understand that it's a lot more responsibility. You have to cook and clean. You have to get yourself up and on the bus in the morning. You have to shop for food and do laundry."

"I don't mind," Jillian said. And in truth, she didn't. She'd been talking about moving out for months. In Jillian's mind, the transition from "I wide bike" to "I'm ready for my own place" was small and seamless. When she determines she wants to do something, there is no dissuading her.

Kerry and I had been thinking the same. It was the next logical step. It was the biggest step of all. We'd been working toward it for only the past 21-plus years. A few months after her 21st birthday, Jillian started banging the drum.

"I think your little girl is ready to move out," she announced.

"Is that right, big-time? What makes you think that?" I asked.

"I can count money."

Really?

"Yep. And I can make dinner."

It was true about dinner. Kerry had started giving her recipes to follow. As Jillian proceeded through the steps, Kerry took pictures: The ingredients, aligned on the kitchen counter and then being prepared for cooking. What the finished product looked like. Kerry put the pictures and the recipes in a three-ring binder.

"I make my world-famous meat loaf," Jillian explained.

"That you do," I said.

Early on, Jillian had some trouble reading recipes. Occasionally, measurements threw her. There's a big difference between a tablespoon of salt and half a cup. The nights Jillian cooked, I was ready for just about anything, including a call to the pizza guys.

But Jillian learned. She'd begun helping me on the grill: Salmon, turkey burgers, hot dogs. Jillian's capabilities extended to spaghetti and meatballs and baked chicken. Her repertoire was far more extensive than mine was at age 21. If it didn't fit in a Crock-Pot, I didn't eat it.

"There's more to moving out than cooking," I said.

"I do my own laundry," Jillian shot back. Actually, she did some of her laundry, occasionally. Jillian was still a little shaky when it came to water levels and temperatures. And she needed a stepstool to reach the knobs on the washing machine and dryer.

"Yeah, you do laundry. Once every three months."

"Dad."

"Jillian, if we let you do laundry only when you wanted, you'd walk around looking stricken," I noted. "Child Services would come after us."

"Da-a-a-a-d."

Every couple of days after that, Jillian tossed out some form of moving-out pronouncement. We could be discussing the fate of the free world or where to find a good $5 cigar, and Jillian would interject, "I'm not your little girl anymore."

"You'll always be my little girl."

"What I mean is, I'm ready to move out."

We'd started to make a plan. With Ellen and Dimitri, Kerry and I set fall 2012 as the target time. We picked September, which would coincide hopefully with the start of Jillian and Ryan's last year at Northern Kentucky. We didn't want to combine the stress of their finding jobs with the strain of living on their own. A year of having the certainty and regimentation of college would ease the transition. We didn't tell Jillian and Ryan this. They still had to learn some things.

Managing money, eating properly, keeping an apartment

relatively clean, and not bothering the neighbors. And, ah, well, um . . . sex.

They would share a bed and all the typical urges. It would be wrong to assume that adults with disabilities don't have the same desires as the rest of us. Jillian and Ryan experience the same culture. They go to the same movies, watch the same TV shows, and absorb the same obsessions. They're curious, too.

We had to take this in stages. We didn't dismiss their capacity for love or their understanding of the different ways to express it. We encouraged it. But those with intellectual disabilities bloom late on the emotional side, too. Things needed to be explained. Things needed to be tried.

The first step was to leave Jillian home alone for a night. Not long after Jillian's 21st birthday, in October 2010, Kerry and I spent the night at a local hotel, ten minutes from the house. We checked in late in the afternoon. We armed Jillian with copious Post-it notes—lock all the doors, don't answer the land line, feed Lucy—a box of spaghetti, a bag of frozen meatballs and one request: "If you get scared, you can call."

Jillian did call that night, at 8:30 p.m. or so. I could hear music in the background. "What are you doing?" I yelled into the cell phone.

"I'm having a great time," she said.

She'd cooked dinner, cleaned the kitchen, and made popcorn. She planned on watching a movie. For the moment, she was listening to music and singing loudly. "You okay?" I asked.

"Yes, I am. You guys stay as long as you want."

Well, all right then.

That test aced, Jillian assumed she was ready for bigger things. "I'll stay with Ryan," she declared.

Well. That would take more prep work.

We'd started a few years earlier, when Jillian was 19 and Ryan was 21—by encouraging them to spend time alone after dates. The basement was the room of choice. We'd give them an hour or two. No rules about keeping lights on, or feet on the floor. We'd had The Talk. Actually, we'd had several. They were the same talks we'd had with Kelly, covering the same, well-worn ground. Ellen and Dimitri did the same with Ryan.

All agreed Ryan would be respectful of Jillian's wishes. She would drive the bus when it came to what sort of mutual exploring would be done, and when. Ryan, being a guy, was frisky. Jillian, not being a guy, was less so. Each was persistent.

On a drive to NKU one morning, Jillian was riding shotgun, with Ryan in the back. He leaned forward to drape one arm over her left shoulder. He curled his other arm around the back of the seat and across her right shoulder.

Ryan was holding a picture of the two of them from a prom they'd attended. He rested his chin on her shoulder and extended the photo to where Jillian could see it. In the picture, they're holding hands. "I love you, honey," Ryan said. Jillian returned the kindness. Then Ryan said, "Is this how you're going to hold my hand when you're pregnant?"

I swerved into the adjacent lane.

"Not yet, Ryan," Jillian said.

"Honey," Ryan said. "Come on."

"That ain't happenin'," Jillian said.

Order restored, I caused no accidents. And Jillian and Ryan set out on that timeless road of appropriate and respectful intimacy.

That didn't end the discussion, though. Kerry and I knew that, at some undetermined time, we would have to sit down with Ellen, Dimitri, Jillian and Ryan, and explain to them that they wouldn't be having children. The likelihood of a couple with Down syndrome having a child with Down syndrome is great. Even if it weren't, the responsibility of caring for a child would be overwhelming for them. That was a topic for a future time.

Meantime, Kerry had a woman-to-woman talk with Jillian. Intimacy confused Jillian. It came with all the typical human emotions. When do I allow it? When I do, what do I allow? How much is too much? These were delicate negotiations, even for a couple whose entire dating lives had been spent with each other.

"When you're ready, you'll know," Kerry said.

"I'm not ready yet," Jillian responded.

Kerry said there was nothing wrong with that. "Ryan loves you and respects you. He understands."

"Okay, Mom."

Less than a week later, we were all at our cabin in the woods, a weekend place 70 miles away that we'd built a decade earlier. Ellen and Dimitri owned a place just up the road so Ryan had also made the trip. He and Jillian had taken a long walk together before dinner, apparently engaging in high-level talks. They both arrived back at the cabin, pleased with themselves.

" 'Member that talk we had last week?" Jillian asked Kerry.

Yes.

"I'm ready now."

That's when we arranged for Ryan to spend the night at our house. It was almost a year after Kerry and I left Jillian home alone. This time, Kerry and I would be staying at the cabin. Jillian and Ryan would make dinner together, watch a movie, have dessert and . . .

As Kerry and I were leaving, I said, "Ryan?"

"Yes, sir?"

"You be good to my little girl." *Whap-whap-whap*.

"I've always been treating your daughter good, sir," he said.

We spent a few hours on the deck at the cabin that night, wondering what the lovely couple was doing at that very moment, and marveling a little at the human condition.

"Can you believe this?" I asked Kerry.

Silly question. Kerry had been the one who'd always assumed Jillian would attend typical classes, take college courses, get her own place to live and get married.

"Of course I can," she said. "But do you think she's ready?"

"No idea," I said.

How do any of us know? Having sex is one thing. Making love is something altogether different. One is a motel room; the other is a wedding night. Virginity is quaint now, damned near Victorian. The notion of "saving" oneself for marriage probably died with the invention of the backseat. Were Jillian and Ryan ready? Only they knew that.

I knew one thing, though: Their first time would be all it was supposed to be. It wouldn't be cheap or regretful. They'd come too far for that. Jillian was appropriately concerned; Ryan was entirely respectful. They'd been together seven years. They knew each other very well. Knowing each other intimately didn't seem a great leap.

Ellen summed it up best: "They are there for each other, so they don't have to do things alone. Things the rest of us do, that have to seem so scary for them. They're moving forward together, knowing that each loves the other totally for who they are."

We resisted calling them, except once to see how they were doing. They were doing fine. Okay, then. Goodnight.

We got home the next afternoon, not knowing what to expect and ready for just about anything. The lovely couple was sitting in the family room. Canary-eating cat grins dominated their gazes.

"How was it?" Kerry asked.

"Good," Jillian answered.

I cocked my head and raised my left eyebrow, a move Ryan had long since termed "The Look." Fist found palm. *Whap whap whap.*

I pretended to be greatly concerned. At least I think I pretended.

"*How* good?" I asked.

"Dad," Jillian said.

"Paul," Kerry said.

"I'm always good to your daughter, sir," Ryan said.

And that was that.

Later, Kerry sat Jillian down. "I want you to be able to tell me things," she started. "I want to know what you're thinking and feeling. I don't want you to think you can't talk to me. We're both women. We understand these situations. I want you to be comfortable talking to me. Okay, Jillian?"

Jillian nodded. Yes.

"Good. Is there anything you'd like to say?" Kerry asked. "Any questions you have? I want this to be a wonderful experience for you. This will just be between us. I promise. So?"

"I have just one question," Jillian said.

"Anything," Kerry said, anticipating the best, prepared for everything, grateful to be included. This was a titanic moment. "Anything at all. What?"

"When can we do it again?"

They would do it again, many times, before the move. Sleep in the same bed, that is. What transpired there was their business. We never asked. On vacation, they slept in the same bed, listening to the waves of the Atlantic outside their window of a house in St. Augustine, Florida. Dimitri bought them a book. It contained, well, helpful hints, fully illustrated. They stopped wanting to go to the cabin.

"Ryan and I stay home," Jillian offered.

From the cabin, Kerry and I would call once at night, and again in the morning. The a.m. calls were especially amusing. Once, Kerry called Jillian's cell, then the home phone, and got no answer on either. She left messages on each. We worried briefly until Jillian called back.

"Sorry, Mom. We didn't hear the phone."

We?

"Ryan and I," Jillian said. "We were in the shower."

Oh.

JILLIAN STILL WASN'T EXACTLY sure about things. The day before her appointment with the gynecologist, in June 2012, when the doctor would prescribe birth control pills, Kerry prepped her. "You'll have to tell the doctor you sleep with Ryan," Kerry said. Jillian nodded, warily.

"You'll want to tell her you two are getting your own apartment, probably in the fall, and eventually you will have intercourse."

"In-course?"

"Sex. I assume you haven't yet," Kerry said.

Jillian said no, they hadn't.

"Why not?"

"Because I'm not ready," Jillian said.

"What worries you about having sex?"

"I don't want to have a baby yet," Jillian said.

"Perfect, because that's what the Pill is for." Sex isn't just about having babies, Kerry told her. "It's fun. Is Ryan ready?"

"Yes," Jillian said. "He wants to have a baby."

"Well, you're not ready to have a baby. You are ready to have sex, whenever you feel like it," Kerry said.

Jillian gave that a long thought. "We're going to have a dog," she said.

Once we told Jillian and Ryan we were targeting September for their move, they talked about nothing else. We'd taken Ryan with us on vacation to Florida. On the way back, Kerry and I overheard this conversation:

Jillian: "You don't have to tell me now. You just think about it and tell me later. But I need to know because we're going to live together forever."

Ryan: "Honey, I don't know if I have any allergies."

They were never allergic to each other. They fought, of course, usually when Ryan flirted with other girls or Jillian got too bossy. (She got that from her mother.) They worked it out.

They wouldn't have lasted seven years if they hadn't behaved maturely and respectfully.

Moving out, moving in, the mysteries of attraction, the intimacy involved. Jillian's fearlessness was put to the test. Until then, her life had been safely cocooned. She knew where her heart was. It was at home, with her brother, her parents and her dog. It would be moving now. It would take up residence with her boyfriend, in a place of their own—where they could stay up late, but she couldn't say goodnight to her parents.

Kids move out all the time. The scene is played out a million times a day. Not so much for young adults who have Down syndrome.

The push-pull got to Jillian occasionally. After the talk we'd had with her on that night in May 2012, she excused herself. "C'mon Lucy," she said and walked through the house and out the front door. Lucy followed.

Jillian sat on the front stoop for an hour. She put her arm around her dog. I don't know what Jillian was thinking—weighing the pros and cons, probably. I liked it, though. Jillian was assessing her life and where it was going, just like the adult we'd always hoped she'd be. I was proud of her.

CHAPTER 30

One More Drive

Into a dancer you have grown.
—JACKSON BROWNE

Seventeen years earlier, when I put Jillian on that first school bus and watched her attack its steps on her knees, I'd hoped for this moment. Now the moment was here, and I didn't know what to do. Yearning is the most contrary of emotions.

It is a Friday in September 2012. The next day, Jillian will be moving with Ryan into their own apartment, just across the street from the Metro bus stop where for the last three years Jillian has boarded the first of two buses to NKU. Today I will drive Jillian to the bus stop for the last time. It is the final leg of this middle journey between what we've dreamed and what we're realizing. It won't be the last stepping out. Worlds remain for Jillian to conquer, and she can't do it alone. But there is a finality to this one, as if we've run out of sidewalk.

"Are you okay, Jills?" I ask as we get in the car for the eight-mile ride to the bus.

"I'm just a little bit shaky, a little bit," she says.

You and me both.

"It's okay," I say. "Lots of people leaving home for the first time feel that way. Lemme ask you something."

"Yeah?"

"Every time you've done something new, hasn't it worked out okay?"

"Yeah."

"Like your first day at NKU. Remember how nervous you were?"

She nods yes.

"How'd that work out?"

She smiles. "Good," she says.

"Remember your first night home alone, when Mom and I went to the hotel? That worked out great, didn't it?"

"Oh, yeah," she said slyly. "And then me and Ryan started staying home together."

"Ryan and I," I say.

"Da-a-a-a-d."

"Jillian, every time you've done something new—new school, new job, now your own place—it has worked out. That's because you're confident and strong. Right?"

"I'm strong."

The car trips—first to NKU, then to the bus stop—were the logical extension of the breakfast table talks, the Coffee Song and the hand holding. The whole Jillian-Dad catalog. We figured out the world, day after week after year. One passage ended, the next began. I paused to lament the passing of each, but not for long because I knew another would take its place.

Now, I've run out of anothers.

A few days earlier, Missy Jones had told me that in a class she taught about family relationships, Jillian had spent much of the time in tears. Jillian had recounted in great detail our hand-holding days to the school bus stop at the end of the common drive. Now she wasn't crying. At least not a lot.

"Jills, Mom and I won't be far away. Ellen and Dimitri will be even closer. Any time you want us to come over, we will. In the meantime, you get to spend more time with the love of your life. Okay?"

"Okay, Dad," she says. "I'm going to miss you and Mom," Jillian says. "And Lucy."

I know.

"And Dad?" she says.

"Yep."

" 'Member when you held my hand to the bus stop every day?"

"Of course I do," I say.

"I was your little girl then."

"You'll always be my little girl."

"That's what I want to say to you, Dad. I always be your little girl, even now that I have my own place."

"Well, I'm glad that after all these years you've finally wised up," I say.

"You're my best father," Jillian says.

It's a little before 8:00 a.m. when we pull into the parking lot. The bus arrives at 8:05, without fail. Jillian likes to stand at the stop. It makes her feel more grown up. We don't linger. Not even on this day.

"I'm going, Dad," Jillian says.

I know.

"Have a great day, sweetie," I manage.

"I will."

She hugs me, a second or two longer than normal. Or maybe I'm just imagining that. Probably, I am. I watch my almost 23-year-old little girl make the short walk from the parking lot to the bus stop. Time for a new sidewalk.

This constant push-pull occurs with all our children. Pain and pride swirl and dance until they become interchangeable. It hurts so good. We want them to stay. We know they can't. The heart is insistent. It must be ignored.

It's Jillian's life now. Not mine.

I pull from the lot. Three years earlier, I'd have stayed until the bus arrived. That lasted until Jillian allowed that people riding the Metro don't require their parents to hang out until the bus shows up. I drive away.

Jillian stands at the stop. Her backpack tugs at her shoulders. Maybe that's why she appears to be slumping. Maybe it's something else.

I wave as I make the right turn from the lot and toward home. "Bye," I say, through the open car window. She can't hear me. The traffic drowns it out. I say it again, anyway. Goodbye, Jillian.

It's possible to be devastated and overjoyed, all at once.

I punch up Jackson Browne on the Pandora. There are no coincidences in life. Fate is fate. "For a Dancer" is the first tune:

> *Keep a fire burnin' in your eye*
> *Pay attention to the open sky . . .*
> *Into a dancer you have grown.*

I drive home to a house that is suddenly larger and less joyous. Just as it is meant to be.

Three days later, on Monday morning, I call Jillian at 7:50 a.m. I am standing in that nowhere/everywhere place between sad and elated that I think only dads and daughters can know.

"You at the bus stop?"

"Yes, I am," she says.

"Well. Have a great day," I say.

"Oh, I will," Jillian says. "I'm so happy."

CHAPTER 31

Vanuatu

*We have food. No one goes hungry. We have a close
family. I have a girlfriend and the beach. What else
do you need in the world?*
—A NATIVE OF ST. LUCIA, TO
VIDEOGRAPHER TONY MARTIN,
IN *ISLANDS* MAGAZINE, MARCH 2011

If you love someone, they'll love you back.
—JILLIAN

A week after I dropped Jillian at the bus stop for the last
time, I was on an airplane, headed to a football game. Being
trapped in a 737 is a good time to sleep or ponder or do nothing at all. I was about to do nothing when I spotted the top of
a magazine in the seat pocket: *Islands*.

My periodical tastes run narrow: *Time* for news, *Sports Illustrated* for sports. The occasional *Esquire* or *Gentlemen's*

Quarterly for a fix of masculine prose. Magazines like *Islands* don't get my dime because I'm not someone who owns a yacht. The trendiest beachfront bars on Jost Van Dyke aren't even in the daydream bucket.

I am a sucker for escapism though. I dream of cabins in the woods and toes in the sand, curling local beers while pondering nothing as weighty as the next five minutes. I am an idyllist, staring at that Meyerowitz photo, wondering what's beyond the door.

Kerry and I did spend our 20th anniversary in a bungalow high in the hills of St. John, above the rapturously named Chocolate Hole, and number 25 adjacent to Smuggler's Cove on Tortola, in a house that could have been on the cover of, well, *Islands* magazine.

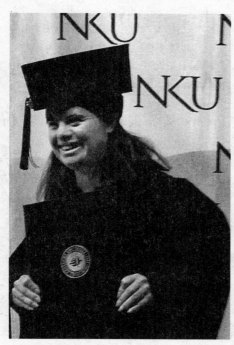

Jillian receives her certificate, during graduation ceremonies at Northern Kentucky University.

So what the hell. I open the magazine, and the first page I find has a headline that asks: "Is This the Happiest Place on Earth?"

It's a story about Vanuatu, a strand of 83 islands and 220,000 souls in the South Pacific where the per capita income is slightly more than $3,000 a year. In 2011, something called the New Economics Foundation, a London-based think tank, decreed Vanuatu happiness to be superior to the everyday version. Vanuatuans—"ni-Vans" to the locals—get the nod because they "are satisfied with their lot, live long and do little damage to the planet."

The author asks a ni-Van why this is so. "They don't know troubles the way you know troubles." Ni-Vans, she says, "put people ahead of things. We measure wealth not by what you keep, but by what you give away. The richest man in Vanuatu is the man who can give away the most pigs."

As another ni-Van says, "We are not so impatient. Here, it is about family." The story expounds on notions of trust, love and spiritual well-being. Ni-Vans live essential lives, defined by core virtues. They don't get snagged on life's muddy periphery. It helps that they live in a place most of us would consider in the Top 10 on the Paradise List. People travel thousands of miles to visit spots like Vanuatu for a few days of sand, sun and good vibrations. It's not a sad life on Bali Ha'i.

Climate is superficial, though. Geography doesn't define well-being or explain it. Paradise would be a barren place if not shared.

Jillian could live on Vanuatu. She could be a ni-Van. She knows what they know. Jillian loves unconditionally and universally. She trusts those close to her. Her schedule is complex—Jillian's social and school calendar is full—but her life is not complicated. The junk that clutters our days—anger, anxiety, jealousy, finances, cynicism, guile, agendas—has no place in her world.

Her concerns are defined by who she loves, and who loves her. Is everyone around her okay?

Jillian is not simple. I do wonder, though, if her disability has blessed her with an ability to fix on essences. One of the worst things you can say about my daughter is also one of the most accurate. I hear it all the time: "These kids are so loving."

I can almost feel the pat on Jillian's head.

These kids?

Compared to whom? *Those* kids?

Being "loving" is not yet a disability trait. It's not compensation. God help us when it is. I'd like to think Jillian would be a fine human being, even without the 47th chromosome. If your daughter's a blond beauty queen, do people assume she's stupid? A cynical world looks at happy and uncomplicated people as unknowing. Jillian knows things.

But more than that, she feels. Down syndrome did not bestow her with the authentic grace and compassion with which she navigates her days. Her natural empathy wasn't genetically arranged. Happiness isn't a tradeoff for her inability to process Algebra II.

Most of life is hieroglyphics. Jillian gets the big parts right. Who loves her, whom she loves. The energy to be optimistic, the effort to be kind. Jillian sees only your good. I want to be more like that. Who doesn't?

Jillian is happy. She's the happiest person I know and would be if she lived in Vanuatu or on an ice floe.

I wonder where Jillian's niceness comes from. It's not genetic. Kerry's nice, but not to an extreme. Kelly is nice because he takes after Kerry. No one has ever accused me of being nice. Jillian's niceness? I can't explain it. It's like explaining what water tastes like. I learn from Jillian's niceness. I hope that being exposed to it causes some of it to take. I'd like to think I can be nice by association.

I'd like to find all mornings in the great shape Jillian finds them. Monday is her favorite day. Monday means a whole new week of fine possibilities. "I love my school," she says, ten months of the year. "I love my job," she says, the other two months.

I'd like to dress my days in the sort of optimism Jillian takes for granted. Happiness isn't a choice for her. It just is. Jillian owns a first-time innocence, all the time.

We've spent 23 years trying to get the world to see Jillian, rather than simply look at her. Seeing opens doors. It's how all of us should regard the world. Jillian comes by it naturally. She sees everything.

Her heart is generous because it isn't cluttered with accessory concerns. Jillian's heart is her gatekeeper. I can't tell you why. Her brain is equally active. She broods and grieves. Her teenage moodiness arrived after she turned 20. Another example of being developmentally delayed, I suppose.

But nothing invades her intellect without approval from her emotion.

"How's Grandpa's heart doing?" Jillian might ask.

Kerry's father had undergone bypass surgery to clear a valve that had been 90 percent blocked. Jillian's question would have been acutely relevant had Sid's operation been last week. It was five years ago.

"His heart is fine, Jills," I say.

She still misses Uncle Pete, a sentiment she revives every

few months. Pete Tranelli was Kerry's uncle. He was the most easygoing of men, the kind of guy who really would pluck a quarter from behind your ear. Jillian sensed his gentleness. He was a favorite of hers, and vice versa. Pete passed a decade ago.

"I still miss my uncle Pete" is what Jillian says about that.

Compassion has a standing reservation at Jillian's table— especially for anyone who has endured physically. My mother had a knee replaced several years ago, and it's not unusual for Jillian to ask: "How's Grandmother's knee doing?" My dad has had circulation issues in one of his legs. Jillian: "How's your dad's leg?"

I've had back problems on occasion. They're aggravated by sitting for long periods of time, usually behind the wheel of a car. When I drove Jillian to the Metro bus stop every morning, she would slide her hand between my seat and my lower back and do what she could to rub out the knots. Even if I currently didn't have any.

"Jillian, my back hasn't hurt for a month," I might say.

"Just making sure," she'd answer.

These aren't occasional bits of conversation. Jillian does this every day. If she sees Nancy Croskey, she'll ask about her two children and her husband. One of my golf buddies was out of work for several months. During that time, whenever Randy's name came up, Jillian would ask if he'd found a job.

Lots of us engage this way. The difference is that Jillian isn't making small talk. She cares about the answer and the people involved. I've asked people those same questions and five minutes later, had no recollection of their response. Jillian's curiosity is real. She either isn't interested in pretend niceties, or she lacks the capacity. Regardless, Jillian isn't wily enough to fake concern.

Her innocence is a by-product of her disability. I'll yield to that generalization. Jillian lacks the intellectual capacity to grasp a lot of what's dangerous in the world. Her stresses are minimal. Her circle is tight. It includes her family, her boyfriend, her dog, her school and her job. They're all good. They rarely disappoint. While she's acutely aware of our stresses, and reacts to them, that is owed to her sensitivity, not her intellect.

Times when Kerry and I have suffered through routine arguments over mindless things, Jillian has asked us if we're getting divorced. "I don't want to lose you guys," she has said.

Her compassion is especially acute when it comes to pets. We've lost pets; all families do. As with everything else, though, Jillian's authentic emotion has made us all feel more deeply.

Every family goes through its share of incidental pets. These aren't the pets that show up in the vacation video or the family portrait. They're the pets you get because you think your child should have a living thing to take care of. Decades later, you're not wistfully recalling your first turtle. You don't take incidental pets for a walk or, if you're Jillian Daugherty, use them as both pillow and mode of transportation, the way she did our dog. No one gives his kid a goldfish for Christmas.

Kelly had multiple goldfish. None lived in the luxury of an actual tank, with a filter and aeration and colored gravel. They hung out in a bowl of tap water. We changed the water every day and fed the inhabitants as instructed. They all died within a few weeks. We didn't especially miss them.

Jillian had Jake, the guinea pig. Jake was incidental in that he didn't relate to us in any meaningful way. Jake liked to eat. He'd express pleasure when he knew food was coming. Beyond that, we were scenery.

Kelly once tortured his little sister with a diabolical scheme to test Jake's aerodynamics. "How do you think Jake would look in a parachute?" he asked her. The plan was to outfit Jake in a custom-tailored sandwich bag, wrap it (and him) in string and throw him out Jillian's second-floor bedroom window. The plan stalled when Kelly couldn't properly attach the string to the bag. Or Jake to the string. Otherwise, young Jake would have had an early demise.

Jake didn't get out much, because when he did, he ran and hid and that made Jillian cry. Jake spent most of his life in a glass box. He was on extended incidental time, to everyone but Jillian. Jillian loved Jake.

That's why it hurt to tell her Jake had passed on. We gathered our courage and knocked on Jillian's bedroom door. She was 11 years old at the time. Jake was 3. "Come in," she said.

"Jake's dead," we told her.

"No, he's not," Jillian said.

"He died last night. Remember how he was coughing a lot?" Jake had developed some sort of wicked guinea pig asthma. At least that's what we diagnosed. We didn't take Jake to the veterinarian because, well, he was a guinea pig.

"Jake's in heaven now," we said.

"When's he coming back?" Jillian wanted to know.

Jillian insisted we give Jake a proper burial, so we wrapped him in a hand towel and placed him in a shoe box. We forced a shovel into the frozen ground in the backyard. When the hole was sufficiently deep, Jillian lowered the box and said some things that needed saying.

"I'll miss you, Jake. I love you. Even though you're dead, you're still a good boy."

We all agreed.

Eleven years later, in random moments, Jillian will offer, "I really miss my guinea pig."

Her first dog was Walker, a huge black Labrador retriever we got when Jillian was five years old. Walker was not a dedicated lover of all things people. She owned a cat's personality. Walker made you earn her affection. She got along great with Jillian, though. Walker allowed Jillian to use her back as a mattress. She was okay with Jillian riding her around the yard. Some winter nights, Walker would disappear. After a few instances of frantically canvassing the house, we learned that Walker could be found at the bottom of Jillian's bed, completely under the covers.

But Walker wasn't completely passive. Until the age of five, when she blew out a knee terrorizing the neighbor's Dalmatian, Walker was a lunatic. She jumped through every window screen on the first floor. She left skid marks on the tender, early spring grass. She excavated the yard, seeking moles. Walker wasn't obedient. She didn't come when you called, unless meat was involved. She didn't sit or do tricks. She lived a decade without doing anything she didn't want to do.

She sensed Jillian's gentleness, though. She let Jillian abuse her with abandon.

Walker lived her last days motionless on our driveway, eyes open to the world she once ruled and riled. Her liver was shot.

Jillian knew something was up. She was 15 years old by then and had seen Jake and her uncle Pete leave. She was familiar with the permanence of death. She'd walk out to the driveway and sit with Walker for long stretches of time.

"I don't want to lose my Walky-dog," she'd say.

We waited for Jillian to go to school before we helped Walker from the driveway and took her to the vet for the last time.

There is a higher heaven for dogs. It's entirely uncomplicated by baser human emotions. Dogs are nicer than people. They elicit our best intentions. They teach us things, but the instruction never sticks. Their love is unconditional. We love them back.

The vet injected Walker with a lethal dose of anesthetic. Kerry and I rubbed the fur on her back and said our goodbyes. Jillian was at lunch in the school cafeteria.

Later, she would note Walker's absence by saying, "The floor is empty."

Jillian feels. For all the right reasons. She understands that a significance of death is that it reminds us how good it is to be alive. She cried buckets when Jake died. She thinks of him still. She has a new dog now, Lucy the golden retriever. Lucy is eight years old. At random moments, Jillian will announce her love for Lucy, with an asterisk: "But I still miss my Walky."

The soul is an engine that hums by spirit and feel. It works best when the heart is aligned and in tune. Walker was a good soul, and she recognized a kindred spirit. Maybe Walker misses Jillian too.

It seems callous to compare Jillian to a beloved family pet, and maybe it is. But when we seek companions with the qualities Jillian possesses, we don't often find them in other humans.

Libraries and bookstores are weighted with books about What Really Matters. We seek wisdom on loving, coping, relating and doing better. It's not a cottage industry. It's more of a mansion.

Could it be the answer is right in front of us? Or right in front of me? The five-year-old asking to hold my hand as we walk to the bus stop for her first day of kindergarten. The young lady seeking my assurance as she descends the stairs to greet her date for that first Homecoming dance. *Yes, Jills, you are beautiful. And nervous is okay.*

In April 2011, Jillian had a rough morning. She still gets congested when the pollen rolls in. The mucus makes its way from her nose to her lungs. When it backs up, she vomits. It happens several times a year, a remnant, maybe, of those 11 days spent in the hospital as a six-week-old, when the mucus nearly suffocated her.

She spent the morning bent over a trash can in her bed. "I'm sorry I'm sick," she said.

I rubbed her back some. I told her to lie down and relax. "Maybe the yucky stuff will calm down if you do," I say.

"I hate my nose," Jillian says.

I brought her some toast and rubbed her back a little more. "I'm sorry, sweetie," I say. Then I walk out and close the door behind me. Later, Jillian improves enough to go to the YMCA for a workout. In the car, she says this:

"I miss my father-daughter time."

"Me, too," I manage.

"We still in love, Dad," she says. It's a statement, not up for debate.

"Yes, we are," I say.

"If you love someone, they'll love you back."

"So," I say, "I took care of you this morning, and you love me?"

" 'Zackly," Jillian says.

I wish I had Jillian's heart. I'd like to love unconditionally. Heart quakes, unprompted. I'd settle for knowing what that feels like. How is it to trust without fear and to live without guile? It must be like flying, only freer.

I'll probably never get to Vanuatu. I can read about it, though, in a magazine on an airplane eight miles high while flying across the tissue of earth's atmosphere. I can experience it, too. Jillian is in the passenger seat. She leans over and offers a hand in the small of my spine.

"How's your back feeling?" she asks.

CHAPTER 32

Moving Day

The bird cage is empty.
Yeah, but the trees are full.
—OPIE TAYLOR AND HIS FATHER, SHERIFF
ANDY TAYLOR, ON *THE ANDY GRIFFITH SHOW*

You can't live your life in a day. You can only feel as if you have.

The apartment was just across the street from the Metro stop. It was five minutes from Ellen and Dimitri and ten minutes from us. It was convenient: The happy couple could walk to the supermarket, the sports bar and the discount department store. This was a fine perk, given that they didn't drive and their legs were short.

It was an older, established complex, rambling and leafy, filled with two-story units, attractive to young, single professionals. It had a fitness center, where the couple could take classes. The clubhouse bar had nightly happy hours. In the summer, the bar opened to the swimming pool and hot tub. Parties were the norm.

We found a one-bedroom apartment for Jillian and Ryan on the second floor, at the far edge of a cul de sac. Their deck overlooked woods and a pond. It resembled a treehouse.

They both agreed it was a fantastic place to begin a life together.

"Awesome," Ryan said.

"My dream house," said Jillian.

The day was all business. We had known this day was coming. We'd planned on it. The actual move was just a formality. It was a lifetime achievement award.

We recruited Ellen's brother, Ryan's uncle Rick, who owned an ancient pickup truck. We hauled Jillian's queen bed from her room at our house, the same room where the moon had etched a silver ribbon across her face 22 years earlier. We donated a kitchen table and chairs. We packed her life into cardboard produce boxes we got from the grocery store. Books, photos, CDs, journals, movies. Pieces of what had defined her, placed neatly in rows.

Jillian took a chair and her laptop and a few things to hang on a wall. She took a framed poster of the NKU men's basketball team. And that was it.

We dropped off the bed at the apartment. The satellite TV man was there, installing. We drove the five minutes to Ryan's, where we hauled an armoire down a flight of stairs. We loaded a new couch and a used coffee table into the bed of the truck and tied it all down. We drove back to the apartment, lugged everything upstairs and set it all up.

It's amazing how portable a lifetime can be. The whole move took about two hours.

We gathered around the coffee table and opened a bottle of champagne. The Daughertys and Mavriplises had made a habit of toasting occasions great and small: Homecomings and proms, graduations and college acceptances. Also, simple evenings out or ones spent on the deck in the arms of a summer moon.

Ellen and Dimitri knew what Kerry and I knew: The smallest of greatnesses are always worth cheering.

To Jillian and Ryan and your new lives together.

Everyone spoke. I don't remember what was said. If I'd made more than a cursory toast, I'd have saluted everyone in the room. We'd prepared forever for this day. We'd assumed it would occur. We'd never doubted it. We might have been naïve about the challenges we would face, but our naïveté fueled our optimism, and that optimism guided our lives.

More than two decades earlier, we'd been entrusted with gifts. We knew that then. We know it more on this day. Now we set out to make two lives whole. We wasted no time lamenting or looking back. We'd pushed and prodded and made a nuisance of ourselves. We'd asked that Jillian and Ryan be allowed to define their potential, not have it assigned to them. Everyone has the right to aspire.

We demanded they be seen, not looked at.

We expected it, and we accepted nothing less.

And now, here we were. In their apartment, toasting an idea, and a dream not denied or deferred, but fully alive.

Salud.

"I just want to say, we love you guys, and we'll never forget you," Jillian said.

"Cheers," Ryan said.

Everything builds. This is what Kerry and I took from the day. Jillian the toddler would stumble and fall. We waited for her to pick herself from the floor. We'd make Jillian look people in the eye when she was talking to them. We had her answer the telephone and order her own meals at restaurants.

We wanted her to get lost because those who are never lost can never be found.

In high school, at Northern Kentucky. On campus, on the bus. We were happy, though nervous, when Jillian called from downtown to say she'd missed her connecting bus. That meant she had to figure out her next move. To get to NKU, she needed a Plan B. Failure is a good teacher, but only if you're allowed to fail.

"An opportunity to problem-solve," Kerry called it.

Jillian and Ryan solve problems. They wouldn't have made it to moving day if they didn't.

"They have fights," Kerry said. "But they've learned how to fight. That's important, too. I'm glad they've had fights. They've talked it out, and they're better for it."

Jillian and Ryan have always been a good match. Ryan is book smart. He reads the newspaper every day. He can tell you if the Cincinnati Reds won the night before, and who the Cincinnati Bengals will play on Sunday. He is better than Jillian at the vital everyday: Reading signs and menus, following written instructions.

Jillian is street smart. She is decisive and poised in social situations. Together, they figure things out.

ADULTS WITH DOWN SYNDROME do live on their own. More often than not, they need outside help: Group homes with live-in caregivers, usually, or shared apartments where they receive regular visits from social workers.

Jillian and Ryan weren't blazing a trail, but they weren't far behind the leaders. We assumed they would need help budgeting and planning meals. A certain vigilance would be expected from us.

Turn off the stove and the burners. Don't play your music too loud. Don't leave a log burning in the fireplace when you go to bed. Blow out the candles.

Here's how to use the dishwasher, here's how to re-set the DirecTV after a storm. Here's what to do if you blow a fuse in the bathroom while running the hair dryer. Don't keep spoiled food, don't leave the milk out. Here's how to write a check.

The mechanics of running a household could be taught. As with everything else, it would take a little longer for them. That wasn't important. Ryan and Jillian had the building blocks. They had the fundamentals. That was important. You can't spend five minutes teaching love and trust. Earning respect isn't like changing a lightbulb.

"I can't imagine having a richer life. To them, it's all about love and what really matters," Ellen said. "It's not special. It's just what's good."

"I'm happy to know they are where they should be," Kerry said at the end of moving day.

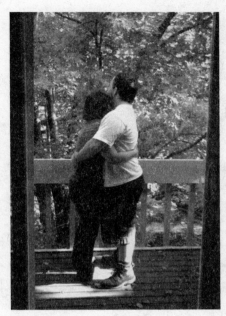

Jillian and Ryan, in their first apartment.

I took a picture of them, just after the toast and before we parents left. Jillian and Ryan stood on their treehouse deck in full embrace. Her arms wrapped around his waist. His arms started at her shoulders and creased her back, his hands locked and forming a V at the base of her spine. They are looking away from the apartment and into the tree branches that hung just a few feet from the railing. They don't know I've trained the camera on them.

It is a blue early-Indian-summer day. A spot of sunshine has snaked its way through the trees, eluding the branches to alight on the floor of the deck, exactly and entirely where Jillian and Ryan have placed their feet.

A Joel Meyerowitz, Cape Light moment, perhaps.

It is their new day, full of its own mysteries, yielding its own endless possibilities. "Goodbye, you guys," we say to them, as we make our way out their door. "Have fun."

The door clicked shut behind us. It seemed to close and open all at the same time.

CHAPTER 33

Number 47

All of us want to do well. But if we do not do good,
too, then doing well will never be enough.
—ANNA QUINDLEN

A few weeks after she was born, we received official word from the geneticist that Jillian did, indeed, have Down syndrome. Jillian owned three copies of Chromosome 21, instead of the usual two. Trisomy 21, it's called, the most common form of Down syndrome.

Human cells contain 23 pairs of chromosomes, 46 in all. This was Number 47. This bit of the-earth-is-round information came with its own sadness. Until then, Kerry and I still held tiny hope the earth would be flat.

Number 47 has, in fact, been king. But not in the way we might have guessed. We knew it would limit her intellectually. We understood that the physical traits it mandated would have permanent social consequences. We were ready to make her life as good as it could be.

We just didn't understand how good Jillian would be. In the literal sense.

If you believe there are no coincidences, you have to at least entertain the notion that Number 47 has a purpose beyond sadness. If you are anything other than terminally pessimistic, you believe the extra chromosome has some beneficial reason for being.

Number 47 contains a lot that makes us good. It has to. Somewhere in that bonus wiring is a connection to compassion and kindness—a plan for how to be better. Number 47 puts out the fires of ego and envy and vanity and guile. It filters anger. Thanks to 47, Jillian lives a life of joy, giving and receiving in equal time. Nothing defines her more. Number 47 isn't a governor on her aspirations. It's an extra storage tank for all her good stuff.

Not long ago, I sat with my mother in the living room of my parents' home in Florida. She was nearing 80 years old when we gathered in the morning to have coffee. We talked about Jillian, as we have lots of times over the years. And my mother said this: "Jillian is the best Christian I know."

Elsye Daugherty isn't devout. She is spiritual. It's an important part of her life and my father's. It isn't an important part of mine. So I asked her, "What does that mean?"

Twenty-three years earlier, a day after Jillian was born, my mother had had a vision of Christ, telling her Jillian would be fine. I've never had a similar experience, nor has anyone else, as far as I know. All our visions have been self-generated. What has come true has been the result of an all-earthly-angels-on-deck offensive, not some assurance from on high.

What does that mean, being the best Christian?

"She's kind," my mother said. "She loves genuinely. She gives. She enjoys life. Do you remember the story you told me about Jillian on the Metro bus?"

I said yes.

I'd gotten an e-mail from a passenger on the bus Jillian rides daily to and from downtown Cincinnati. He knew me because of my job. I'd written about Jillian several times. He wanted me to know some things he saw one winter morning:

> *Paul,*
>
> *Just wanted to send you a quick note. I was in a sour mood this morning when my bus didn't show up so I had to wait an extra 40 minutes in the cold for the next bus to arrive. This bus was packed, standing room only, but a young woman in an NKU sweatshirt gave up her seat to a passenger who just got on the bus. Then, this same young woman offered her coat to someone else on the bus who said she was cold. I overheard someone else talking to her and called her "Jillian." I struck up a conversation with her about school and the NKU basketball team (of which she told me she was a manager). I concluded that I just met your daughter. What a terrific person she is. She brightened the day for me and a few others packed into the bus today because of her kind actions, and I just wanted to pass it along.*
>
> *Mike Herrel*

"That's Jillian," my mother said. "She acts like the rest of the world should act but doesn't."

Jillian not only has those qualities. She inspires them in others. Those who know her are moved to do better, to be better. To do good. We're only as good as the way we treat each other. It's hard not to be good when Jillian is around.

"You and Mom and my brother are my heart," Jillian says. I couldn't tell you when, exactly. She says it a lot.

"What about Ryan?" I ask. "Isn't he your heart, too?"

"Oh, definitely," she says. "Ryan is my favorite boy."

To get to Jillian's heart, simply open yours. If her heart ever breaks, we'll all be lesser for it. Maybe that's what my mother meant.

It's an intrinsic knowing. Knowing what matters, and what to do with it. Knowing the smallest of joys. A hug offered, a smile received. Jillian's knowing isn't learned. It's not inherited. It's innate. It's Number 47 on her shoulder, riding shotgun. Her nearest angel.

Without 47, Jillian isn't Jillian. Maybe she keeps her seat and her coat and for Mike Herrel, the day stays gray. She doesn't change Nancy Croskey's life or Dave Bezold's perspective. Kelly Daugherty doesn't spend an extra hour on yet another analysis of Hemingway.

Without 47, Kerry doesn't get to express her true calling to its fullest. Motherhood satisfies her, but it isn't triumphant. Without 47, maybe I forget the feel of Jillian's hand in mine as we walk to the school bus stop. Maybe I never even notice.

I'm not allowed to take life for granted, not for the last 23 years. Forty-Seven did that for me.

Forty-Seven won't allow Jillian to attend Harvard Law or

complete the Sunday crossword in the *New York Times*. She won't drive a car or bear a child. She will draw the occasional double-glance and misguided wonderment. She will be subject to simple minds and judged by hearts too weak to know.

All this is true and sad and immutable.

Forty-Seven is a soul engine, though. It doesn't quit. It's there every time Jillian asks about Grandpa's heart or misses Uncle Pete. It is front and center in her declarations of affection for people and experiences and life. Forty-Seven is right there, earnest in its simplicity.

If you love someone, they'll love you back.

Anna Quindlen wrote, "All of us want to do well. But if we do not do good, too, then doing well will never be enough."

Jillian bridges the gap between doing well and doing good. Lots of us do well. We have successful careers, we make enough money, we live easily, we enjoy a certain physical comfort. We're not especially tolerant when we don't.

How many of us do good?

A friend of mine once described her grandfather as someone who "lived in quiet appreciation of all that God provided." No one would describe the Jillian Daugherty Show as quiet. But the appreciation part never strays.

That's Number 47 at work, I think. I hope. I believe.

CHAPTER 34

A Dream

He did not know he could not fly;
And so he did.
—GUY CLARK

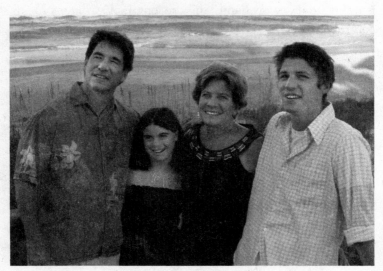

Paul, Jillian, Kerry and Kelly in St. Augustine, Florida.

In the dream, I am flying a box kite on the beach in St. Augustine, Florida, a place where we have spent many family vacations. It is the gentle end to a timeless day, a breezy early evening, clear and a deepening blue. The box kite is adept at handling big winds. On two of its sides are the faces of Jillian and Ryan.

The kite is soaring in the updraft. The faces of Jillian and Ryan are tugging at the string, laughing as they pull away. Higher and higher.

I dream rarely. When I do, I remember only nonsensical shards. But this dream is clear.

I am the keeper of the string. My hands and fingers claim a thrilling ache as they struggle to keep the string taut and the kite rising. I love this kite. I love the way it owns the wind and tempts the heavens as it escapes. It is fearless and yearning. It is limited only by my hands and the length of string my hands control.

Jillian and Ryan appear on the beach, in person, to stand with me as the day's light ebbs. They laugh when they see their likenesses, way up there. They watch me struggle with the kite and the wind. The ache spreads from my fingers and hands to my arms, until all are joined in a collective, thrilling pain. I am Santiago, fighting the marlin.

I run down the beach with the wind. I am fighting the kite, while accepting its needs. The push-pull is comforting and familiar. Jillian and Ryan run alongside, our bare feet in triplicate on the firm, damp sand. They laugh at their likenesses, far above.

The beach is empty, the tide is receding. I stop to catch my breath. As the sun slips below the dunes and toward the marsh and the river beyond, its reclining light paints pastels across Jillian's gaze. It's the same glow from long ago, when she was a baby in her crib and the moon was doing the painting.

So many years pass so quickly. The mantra—expect, don't accept—has done its duty. The battles at school are long since decided. They're monuments in a field, dedicated to all who strive. The aspirations we've had for Jillian have become reality. The race has been run. We will still be here for her. But only when she needs us. Pride and melancholia mix. They feel like my arms and hands. Worthwhile pain as my kite tugs at me, seeking its own place in the sky.

"It's time to let go, Dad," Jillian says.

"No. I still got it." The kite is a dot, but somehow, I still see the faces on it, of Jillian and Ryan. I see them, and it makes me hold on tighter. The ache extends to everywhere. Jillian says, "You need to let it go."

But why? Just a little longer. "I still got it," I repeat.

Ryan says then, "Sir. It's time."

He's right. It's time. I uncurl my cramping hands to unleash the string. The string tears through my fingers and into the air, so quickly. The kite sails away, higher. The faces disappear. When last I see them, they're on the horizon, borne on the wind, laughing and seeking their way.

Jillian and Ryan Get Engaged

I was happy-crying.
—JILLIAN

On the afternoon of December 19, 2013, my cell phone beeped with a message from the estimable Ryan Mavriplis. "Sir," he said, "there is something I would like to talk to you about."

I've known Ryan for nearly a decade, and he still calls me "sir." I know what he wants to discuss. "I would like it if maybe we could go have a beer," he says.

A month earlier, Ryan and Jillian had shopped for a ring setting in which to put a diamond that belonged to Ryan's great-grandmother. They'd been together for more than nine years, the last year of which they'd shared an apartment. It was time.

Ryan's uncle Rick worked in a jewelry store, so the shopping was easy. Ryan was serious that day. His gaze could have cut steel. Jillian, meanwhile, wouldn't have needed a rocket to reach the moon. She could have jumped. She gazed at the display case with eyes like pie plates.

I picked up Ryan at their apartment at 5:30 p.m.

"What do you want to talk about," I asked. "How the Reds are going to do this year?"

"I always take care of your daughter, sir," Ryan said. This was serious business. No time for joking.

"I'm glad about that," I said. "What's on your mind?"

After a big pull on his beer, Ryan got right to the point. "You know I love your daughter, right?"

"Yes, I believe I do."

"And I love her and protect her."

"Thank you."

"She's been my girlfriend for a long time."

"Nine years, yes."

"I would be very happy if you would allow me to marry her," Ryan said.

I said, "Can I get back to you on that?"

"Oh," Ryan said. "Okay." He looked as if I'd backed my car over his foot.

"Ryan?"

"Yes, sir?"

"I'm joking. I'm thrilled you want to marry Jillian. I'd be proud to be your father-in-law."

Then we talked about how the Cincinnati Bengals might do in Pittsburgh that weekend.

It was another of those emotional moments that lacked

emotion. Everything builds, so when the crescendo arrives, it is satisfying, not loud. The little wins along the way were always more telling.

Ryan will make a fine son-in-law. He's bright, open and inquisitive. He puts up with my consistent needling, a skill honed by years of observing athletes in locker rooms. If Ryan can hit my pitches, he's ready for the majors.

I am reminded of a conversation we'd had a few years earlier at the vacation house in St. Augustine.

"Good morning, sir," Ryan said. "What are you doing?"

I was on the laptop, paying bills.

"I'm paying bills," I said.

"What bills are you paying?"

"Credit card bills."

"For this house?"

"No."

"Why?"

"Why what!?"

"Why are you paying bills, sir?"

"Because if I don't, they'll lock me up."

"What does that mean, sir?" Ryan knows what that means. He just wanted to keep talking.

"That means I won't be able to pay for your wedding," I said.

"My wedding?"

"Yeah."

"Well, don't get locked up," Ryan said.

Later that same day, Ryan spied me on the front porch, scribbling notes in the margins of Buzz Bissinger's book *Fa-*

ther's Day. It's about Bissinger's relationship with his son, Zach, who is mentally disabled.

"Why are you writing in your book, sir?" Ryan wanted to know.

"I'm inspired by something, for my book about Jillian," I said.

"I'm gonna be in it, right?" he said.

"Yeah."

"I'm going to be famous, too?"

"Yeah. Fame by association."

"What does that mean?" Ryan asked.

"That means get outta here so I can work."

"Yes, sir," Ryan said. He went back into the house. I heard him tell Jillian, "Honey, I'm gonna be famous."

Some 18 months later, I am returning Ryan's call to my cell phone.

"Got your message," I said.

Ryan and Jillian knew they'd be an item from the very first. Their relationship reflected their worldview. No agendas, no guile. They may be special-needs people, but they had no special needs when it came to romance and commitment.

Thirty years earlier, I had not asked Sid Phillips if I could marry his daughter. I didn't even ask Kerry in any proper way. I'd proposed over the telephone. It was a regretful thing to do.

That would never have occurred to Ryan Mavriplis. He is big on the formal touches. He likes the ceremonies. He never misses a chance to toast an occasion, or shake my hand, or call me "sir." He would do this engagement business right.

The night after I gave him the okay, Ryan bought a bunch

of flowers and put them in a vase on the coffee table of their apartment. Candles glowed on the kitchen table. He made a spaghetti dinner. When Jillian arrived home from her job in the athletic department at Northern Kentucky University, Ryan got down on one knee.

"He was holding something behind his back," Jillian recalled a few months later.

"I gave her a speech," Ryan said. "I said I want to be with you because I love you so, so much. I will protect you. Jillian Phillips Daugherty, will you marry me, please?"

Jillian said yes.

"I was happy-crying," she said.

Some 18 months earlier, Jillian and I sat on the deck of our house, having another talk about her impending move. She happy-cried then, too. Independence is nothing if not competing pulls of the heart. I asked her what she loved about Ryan.

"He can really make a girl laugh," she said. She would say almost exactly the same thing after she accepted Ryan's proposal. "He's funny, he's honest, he's smart."

Their life together isn't guaranteed. There's no way to know if Jillian and Ryan will do any better than the rest of us. They bicker and fight. Ryan isn't always attentive. Jillian can be demanding. If they are different from the rest of us, it is in the elemental focus they bring to the task.

They limit the conversation to what universally applies: Love, respect and trust. I don't know if it's because they lack the intellect to stray from the things that count, or because they don't have the desire. It doesn't matter. They get the big things right: Whom they love and who loves them. It really is that simple.

They're not mean to anyone else. Why would they be mean to one another?

Wedding plans commenced immediately. Jillian and Ryan were married on June 27, 2015, on the stone patio of a rustic lodge in a nature preserve, not far from their apartment. Close to 160 guests bore witness. Each played a role in helping the newlyweds reach this day. The village applauded. And danced.

ACKNOWLEDGMENTS

I would like to applaud all who have taken the time to see Jillian, rather than simply look at her. You have made all the difference.

ABOUT THE AUTHOR

PAUL DAUGHERTY has been a sports columnist for the *Cincinnati Enquirer* since 1994. He has covered nearly every major American sporting event, as well as five Summer Olympic Games. He is the author of *Fair Game,* a collection of his sports columns, and coauthor of books with Chad Johnson and Johnny Bench. He blogs daily at *The Morning Line* on Cincinnati.com. He lives in Loveland, Ohio, with his wife, Kerry.